"Thomas Hanna has written a fantastic book answering questions the experts are only beginning to ask. And he does it in a way that lay people as well as health professionals will find exciting reading, full of entertainment and striking insights."

Dieter Kallinke, M.D.
leading Heidelberg pain specialist

"One of the most profound revolutions in our thinking concerns the fundamental connections between body and mind. Now that we begin to understand something of our inner healing powers, along comes **Somatics** *to give form and shape to our new-found knowledge. We have been blessed by Tom Hanna through the publication of this book."*

Paul DuBois, Ph.D.
Executive Director, Association for Humanistic Psychology

"Somatic education is fortunate to have Thomas Hanna. His newest book, **Somatics,** *marks a new maturity and sophistication in the field he named."*

Michael Murphy
Director, Esalen Institute

"If I could, I would put **Somatics** *in the hands of every neurologist, internist, nurse, psychophysiologic therapist, and clinical psychologist in the country."*

Elmer E. Green, Ph.D
The Menninger Clinic

*"***Somatics** *should be translated into every Western language, and it should be read by all parents and educators."*

Gerda Alexander
founder of Eutony

"The missing link between many doctors and their patients can be rediscovered if both parties understand what **Somatics** *is really about: how wisely and wonderfully we are organized to live a better life than many of us do."*

Mark Schmid-Neuhaus, M.D.
Chief Physician, Munich Health Park

Somatics

Somatics

Reawakening the Mind's Control of Movement, Flexibility, and Health

Thomas Hanna

Director of The Novato Institute
for Somatic Research
and Training

Addison-Wesley Publishing Company

Reading, Massachusetts • Menlo Park, California
New York • Don Mills, Ontario • Wokingham, England
Amsterdam • Bonn • Sydney • Singapore • Tokyo
Madrid • San Juan • Paris • Seoul • Milan
Mexico City • Taipei

The two drawings on pp. 5 and 6 originally appeared in *The Body of Life* by Thomas Hanna, published by Alfred A. Knopf, Inc. copyright © 1980 by Thomas Hanna.

Many of the designations used by manufacturers and sellers to distinguish their products are claimed as trademarks. Where those designations appear in this book and Addison-Wesley was aware of a trademark claim, the designations have been printed in initial capital letters (i.e., Vegemite). The term "Somatic Exercises" is trademarked, and may not be used without the permission of Thomas Hanna.

This book is not intended, nor should it be regarded, as medical advice. For such advice you should consult a medical doctor. If you experience serious or protracted pain during or after Somatic Exercises, then you may have problems other than sensory-motor amnesia, and you should consult your doctor immediately.

Library of Congress Cataloging-in-Publication Data

Hanna, Thomas, 1928–
    Somatics : reawakening the mind's control of movement,
flexibility, and health / Thomas Hanna.
    p.   cm.
    Includes index.
    ISBN 0-201-07979-8
    1. Exercise therapy for the aged. 2. Geriatrics. 3. Sensorimotor
integration. 4. Exercise for the aged.   I. Title.
RC953.8.E93H36   1988   88-905
613.7′1—dc19   CIP

Cover illustration by Dorothea Sierra
Text design and illustrations by Kenneth J. Wilson (Wilson Graphics & Design)
Set in 10-point Palatino by Compset, Inc.

17 18 19 20 21 22-DOC-0100999897
Seventeenth printing, November 1997

This book is dedicated to

ELEANOR CRISWELL

Contents

Introduction

The Myth of Aging

One of the most ancient and famous of riddles is that of the Sphinx: "What is it that has one voice and yet becomes four-footed and two-footed and three-footed?" In Greek mythology, Oedipus provided the correct answer: the human being, who crawls on all fours in infancy, walks on two legs in adulthood, and leans on a cane in old age.

This answers the riddle of the Sphinx. But it does not answer a second riddle that lurks within the first: Why is it that humans, having learned to walk upright, may lose this ability and often end up walking with a cane? Clearly, the presumption is that to grow older is to become crippled. This presumption was accepted in the fifth century B.C. when Sophocles wrote about the Sphinx, but oddly enough it continues to be accepted in the late twentieth century.

"It is obvious," we all declare. "Aging itself causes us to become stiff and aching. From the fifth century B.C. to the twentieth century A.D., as humans become older, they become crippled and infirm. How could it be any other way?"

But there is another way. There is no denying the fact that, as we get older, we usually become stiff, but this does not explain *why* this degeneration should occur. The question remains: What happens during aging to account for this decline? How can scientific medicine, which protects us from infections and organic disorders, extending our life span to 80-odd years, fail to protect us from simple bodily stiffness, aches, and pains? Why do we assume that beyond a certain age—say, thirty—our bodies have already started to decay? We are not even middle-aged yet!

Throughout the centuries the riddle within the riddle remains, just as inscrutable to us today as it was to the Ancient Greeks. At the close of the twentieth century, we are still haunted by the myth that aging means degeneration. We may now live longer, but we do not live better. After so long a time something should have improved. With all that we now know, some new information, some new insight, should have made some sense out of why our bodies seem to break down as they enter middle-age. If we could find out how this breakdown occurs, we might conceivably learn how to prevent it.

Twentieth-century science is slowly groping forward toward a better understanding of the body's deterioration. Hans Selye recognized that physiological diseases could arise from psychological causes, such as stress. This is a "somatic" viewpoint: namely, that everything we experience in our lives is a bodily experience. Moshe Feldenkrais put this viewpoint into action with his method of bodily re-education, Functional Integration. I am pleased to say that my treatment based on the work of both Selye and Feldenkrais has achieved some dramatic results in counteracting the aging process. Human beings, once they advance from crawling on all fours to walking on two, no longer need regress to a limping posture once they become older. That is to say, the bodily decrepitude presumed under the myth of aging is not inevitable. It is, by and large, both avoidable and reversible.

I know this to be true, because I have seen it occur thousands of times. Clients I have worked with during the past 12 years evince changes that are real and lasting. Years later they happily confirm the fact. I confess that 20 years ago I would not have believed possible what I see taking place in my office every day. Even though clients—most of them 30 and older—have heard good things about my work, they first come to me with the same mix of hope and skepticism that I once had. But once we finish working together, they typically tell me, "I had no idea that this was really possible. Having had this problem for years, with nothing to help it, I decided I had to learn to live with it." Then they often add an intriguing remark: "You know, even though I didn't think this was possible, somehow I always thought that it *should* be possible."

A similar thought was expressed by a group of physicians, osteopaths, chiropractors, and physical therapists from Australia to whom I had taught some of these procedures: "You have shown us what we thought we should learn during our training but never did. It is the missing link in health care." One of the physicians attending my class was a distinguished cardiologist, practicing in Sydney. In an article he later wrote about his reactions to the class, he said that what he had learned "has as much potential for understanding the mind-body relationship as Einstein's theory of relativity had for physics."[1]

For 12 years now I have been hearing such statements of confirmation, and I am convinced that everyone can avoid the loss of bodily function which is the curse of growing older. We all know, and probably envy, some people who in their later years seem to have avoided the aging process. There is no reason for our bodies to suffer when most of our life is still before us.

Many people in every generation continue to function actively right up until they die. This is a phenomenon gerontologists have finally recognized. They call it "successful aging."[2] We all know of examples. Some of the most famous people in every epoch have lived to an extended age, still working, thinking, and creating right up to the end. Even Sophocles, who gave us the riddle of the Sphinx, wrote his last play when he was 90.

The fact is that, during the course of our lives, our sensory-motor systems continually respond to daily stresses and traumas with specific muscular reflexes. These reflexes, repeatedly triggered, create habitual muscular contractions, which we cannot—voluntarily—relax. These muscular contractions have become so deeply involuntary and unconscious that, eventually, we no longer remember how to move about freely. The result is stiffness, soreness, and a restricted range of movement.

This habituated state of forgetfulness is called *sensory-motor amnesia* (SMA). It is a memory loss of how certain muscle groups feel and how to control them. And, because this occurs within the central nervous system, we are not aware of it, yet it affects us to our very core. Our image of who we are, what we can experience, and what we can do is profoundly diminished by sensory-motor amnesia. And it is primarily this event, and its secondary effects, that we falsely think of as "growing older."

But sensory-motor amnesia has nothing whatsoever to do with age. It can, and does, occur anytime—from childhood onward. Children who grow up in disturbed family situations, or in other fearful environments such as war, show symptoms of sensory-motor amnesia: sunken chests, permanently raised shoulders, hyper-curved necks. Traumatic accidents or serious surgery in young people can cause the same chronic muscular contractions which in older adults are falsely attributed to aging: for example, scoliotic tilting of the trunk, a slight limp, or chronic undiagnosable pain that never disappears during the remainder of one's life.

The reflexes that cause sensory-motor amnesia are very specific. There are three, and I have named them the *Red Light reflex,* the *Green Light reflex,* and the *Trauma reflex.* They are a crucial part of SMA and round out the enormously important discoveries of Hans Selye and Moshe Feldenkrais. Before discussing the three reflexes, however, it is important that I point out the following facts: (1) The effects of sensory-motor amnesia can begin at any age, but usually become apparent in our thirties and forties; (2) SMA is an adaptive response of the nervous system; and (3) *because SMA is a learned adaptive response, it can be unlearned.*

This is my good news: Sensory-motor amnesia can be avoided, and it can be reversed. You can escape it by making direct and practical use of two abilities that are the unique properties of the human sensory-motor system: to unlearn what has been learned; and to remember what has been forgotten. In Part 3 you will find eight *Somatic Exercises.* These provide a direct and effective way to re-program the sensory-motor system. These exercises are a major discovery. First of all, they erase the primary effects of what is falsely attributed to growing older. Moreover, they are particularly important for people in their thirties, who begin to experience the accumulated effects of the Red Light reflex, the Green Light reflex, and the Trauma reflex. In older people, they actually reverse the process, which has caused so many people to feel stiff and aching.

The ultimate benefit of the Somatic Exercises may likely be found in their application to the physical education of young people. I am convinced that a program of early training in personal sensory awareness and motor control would cause, within the span of one generation, a reversal of the major public health problems—cardiovascular disease, cancer, and mental illness. These claims are far-reaching, but no more so than the false notions of the ill effects of aging that have lasted for millennia. Somatic Exercises can change how we live our lives, how we believe that our minds and bodies interrelate, how powerful we think we are in controlling our lives, and how responsible we should be in taking care of our total being. In fact, as these discoveries relate to our conception of what human beings are and can be, they have broad philosophical implications for understanding the nature of our existence.

I am arguing that sensory-motor amnesia describes a category of health problems that has not been recognized until now. Even so, this category probably accounts for more than half of all human ailments. SMA is a pathology that is neither medical nor surgical, and it cannot be diagnosed or treated within these traditions. It is a somatic pathology, requiring not treatment but education. With case histories and research evidence, this book serves as a practical introduction to the new field of Somatics, which holds that first-person human experience must be considered of equal scientific and medical importance as outside, third-person observation.

Somatics provides us with a way to live under the stressful demands of an urban-industrial environment and still remain healthy—physically and mentally. It helps us understand the tendency—of life in general and of technological societies in particular—to wear down our well-being. There is no need to give in to this blindly as the unavoidable effect of aging; rather, we will meet it with open eyes and overcome it.

The message of this book is, in part, that Oedipus's answer to the riddle of the Sphinx is false, a myth. But there is a larger message, which will become obvious once you have learned about sensory-motor amnesia and its causes: As we grow older, our bodies—and our lives—should continue to improve, right up until the very end. I believe that all of us, in our hearts, feel that this is how life really should be lived.

PART 1

The Stories of
Sensory-Motor Amnesia

The sensory-motor system is a mechanism fundamental to all human experience and behavior. And to understand sensory-motor amnesia is to understand one of the fundamental causes of the malfunctions we have falsely believed to be the effects of aging.

In this section are five typical advanced cases of sensory-motor amnesia, in which damage to the body has built up over the years. In my office I see such cases in various forms every day. If you are observant, you will see them on every street in every city and town in the United States. I estimate that at least three-quarters of adult Americans suffer from sensory-motor amnesia, and almost no one knows what to do about it.

Chapter 1

Barney (42 Years):
The Tower of Pisa

Barney, an insurance executive, was in his forties. For several years he had felt chronic pain in his right side. In addition, he would frequently lose his balance and stumble. When his physician heard his complaint, she ordered X rays, but she saw no obvious deformity. She concluded that 42 vigorous years of wear and tear had caused arthritic deterioration of the hip joint. She told Barney, who was a tall man, that he had arthritis, typical of the aging process, and that he had to learn to live with it. She prescribed aspirin and bed rest on days when the pain was extreme.

Not satisfied with this treatment, Barney went to a chiropractor, who told him that the bones of his lower spine were out of alignment and needed adjustment. He adjusted Barney's spine, but the hip continued to hurt. Barney then went to an acupuncturist, who determined which meridians were involved and inserted needles in the appropriate spots. That relieved Barney's pain, but four days later it came back.

So, with this history, which is typical, Barney presented himself to me. He had heard that I do something unusual called "somatic education," which no one quite understood but which nonetheless was said to be highly successful.

Having heard his story, I wanted to find out where the pain was. Barney pointed to the back of his right pelvis in the area between the hip joint and the sacrum. I felt the area. The line of pain was in the gluteus medius muscle, which extends across the buttocks from the top of the thigh to the back center of the pelvis. It is the muscle that we usually contract when standing on one leg. It braces the leg against the pelvis to maintain stability while we lean over to one side. Barney's hip joint was not painful either to the touch or during movement. It was the gluteus medius muscle that was sore.

I informed Barney that he did not have arthritis, but had a painfully overworked muscle that was sore from constant contraction. "Why did my physician tell me I had arthritis?" he asked. I told him I did not know. I knew that X rays do not show muscle tissue, painful or not. And I knew that it was common for physicians to tell patients suffering chronic and medically incurable pain that they had arthritis and there was nothing to do for it. The ancient myth of aging is firmly embedded in modern medicine.

Now that I knew precisely where Barney's pain was, I asked him to stand directly in front of me with his eyes closed. Barney's entire trunk was leaning almost 15 degrees to the right. Because the bulk of his weight was thus always on his right side, his gluteus medius muscle was always contracted.

As Barney stood there, I felt his left gluteus medius muscle. It was soft and uncontracted. Then I felt the same muscle on the right side. It was hard and contracted. When I felt the muscles of his back, they were similar: The left side muscles were relatively soft and relaxed, whereas the right back muscles were tensed—especially those near the spinal column. The muscles on Barney's right side were chronically contracted, pulling him into a scoliotic curve, so that the added weight of his trunk caused his right gluteus medius muscle to contract constantly—thus the chronic pain and fatigue in the muscle.

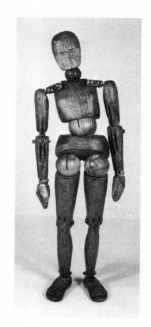

Figure 1
Barney's Posture

Barney could not voluntarily relax the muscles on the right side of his back. They simply would not respond. I had Barney stand in front of a full-length mirror, so that he could see his 15-degree tilt. He had had no idea that he was tilted. But he did remember his physician telling him that his right leg was shorter than his left. We measured his legs, and they were the same length. I asked Barney to bring himself up to a vertical position and then close his eyes. "How does that feel?," I asked. "Are you balanced?"

"No," he said. "I feel tilted to the left." As soon as he relaxed, his trunk immediately tilted back to the right. Then I had him tilt far to the left with his eyes closed and them come back to what he felt was vertical. Without hesitating, he went right back to a 15-degree tilt to the right. "Now I'm vertical," he said. But he looked like the Tower of Pisa.

Not only was Barney's perception of his right side muscles defective, but his perception of his body's position in space was defective as well. His sense of balance was distorted. At one time, earlier in his life, Barney had normal motor control of his muscles on both sides. His senses had been aware of what his muscles were doing to change the posture of his body in space. But he had since lost both his motor control and his sensory awareness. What he once did, he could no longer do. What he once sensed, he could no longer sense. That is the typical effect of sensory-motor amnesia.

I asked Barney if he had ever had any injuries of a serious nature. He said yes, five years earlier he had broken his left thigh in an automobile accident. At that point I knew why he had begun leaning to the right: It is common after leg fractures to tilt one's body to the other side, putting its weight on the leg

that is uninjured. During the long weeks of healing, Barney's right leaning became habituated and totally unconscious. A traumatic accident had brought on
sensory-motor amnesia.

Once Barney was taught how to sense his muscular movements as he once
did, and once he relearned ways to control his muscles, three things occurred:
(1) He no longer had any pain in the pelvis, despite the "arthritis" of old age;
(2) he now stood vertical, with his weight equally balanced on each leg and with
his trunk muscles balanced left and right; and (3) his sense of balance was restored, so that he knew when he was vertical and when he was tilted. He no
longer had the precarious posture that had caused him to stumble constantly.

In brief, Barney no longer had sensory-motor amnesia. And better still, he
now possessed the happy knowledge of how to prevent this from ever occurring
again. He was now self-maintaining, no longer needing my help, nor the help
of any other health professional, to control this problem.

Interlude: **Moving and Feeling—Two Sides of the Same Coin**

When he first came to me, Barney could not properly control the muscles of his
trunk and pelvis—which was a motor deficiency—and could not properly sense
what these muscles were doing with his body—which was a sensory deficiency.
Both problems relate to the central nervous system, that is, the brain and the
spinal cord, which is the overall system that controls the body.

When we look at the central nervous system, we see that the most fundamental aspect of it is that it has, both structurally and functionally, two divisions: a sensory division and a motor division. From the brain down the spine
to the tailbone, the sensory nerves emerge from the back side of the spine and
the motor nerves emerge from the front (see Figure 2).

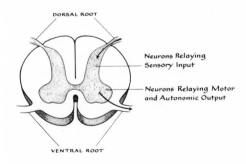

Figure 2
The Sensory and Motor Tract
in the Spinal Cord

Everything we sense in the world outside our bodies and everything we sense inside our bodies comes into our brain by way of the sensory nerves. Everything that we do in the world and every movement we make flows out from our brain down the spine by way of the motor nerves. The sensory nerves control our perceptions of the world and of ourselves. The motor nerves control our movements in the world and inside ourselves by means of their attachments to the muscles of the skeleton and the smooth muscles of the viscera.

These two fundamental divisions of the spinal cord reach upward into the brain: The sensory nerve cells continue to the rear of the central sulcus of the brain, and the motor nerve cells continue to the front of the brain (see Figure 3).

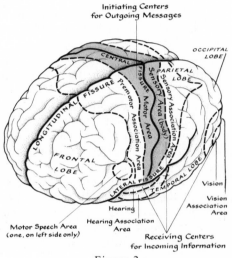

Figure 3
The Sensory and Motor Tract
in the Cerebral Cortex

This structural division is functionally integrated within a single neural system: The sensory and motor functions are two sides of the same coin. In the spine we see the division of the two systems, but in the brain we see their integration.

The sensory nerves carry to the brain information of what is happening in the world as well as in our bodies. Provided with this information, the brain can compute what to do and how to do it: that is, the brain integrates the incoming sensory information with outgoing commands to the motor system. These integrated functions of the sensory and motor systems are so fundamental and so familiar that, like the fish that does not notice the water, we do not notice their ceaseless operation.

We are rarely conscious of these two integrated functions when we do something as simple as turn the pages of a book. When one comes to the end of a page, one's left hand lifts, goes to the right, finds the edge of the next page at the right corner of the book, and turns it to the left. But for the left hand to "find the edge of the next page" demands precise sensory information as to where the hand is and where the book is. When your left hand lifts, it must know where it is going, otherwise it might lift and flop to your side, or hit you in the nose, or go over and touch your right shoulder. Luckily, it doesn't. You know where your hand and book are, because during every instant that you move your hand you are receiving a constant stream of sensory information about the location, direction, contour, trajectory, and speed of the hand movement in relation to the perceived location of the edge of the next page at the right corner of the book.

In contemporary neurophysiological science, the ongoing interplay of sensory information and motor guidance is referred to as a "feedback system" operating in "loops": The sensory nerves "feed back" information to the motor nerves, whose response "loops back" with movement commands along the motor nerves. As movement takes place, the motor nerves "feed back" new information to the sensory nerves about the position of the hand. This feedback loop continues its exchange of information until the hand and fingers touch the page and turn it.

Once we reflect on it, it becomes obvious to us that we require a constant stream of sensory information from the outside in order to maintain ongoing control of our muscular movements from the inside out. We could not purposefully do anything in this world if our sensory-motor system did not constantly function.

To recognize how obviously fundamental the sensory-motor system is to the way we live makes us aware of something else fundamental: If anything goes wrong with the sensory-motor system, our lives will be fundamentally diminished. If something happens that dims our sensory perception, we will not know how to control our bodies and our actions efficiently. If something happens that dulls our motor control, not only will we become limited and inefficient in our actions but our feedback will become confusing and imprecise as well. Inasmuch as the sensory-motor functions are integrated into one system, anything that goes wrong in one part automatically goes wrong with the other. How we sense our world and feel ourselves to be is affected just as much as how we act in the world and how well our bodies function.

Malfunctions of the sensory-motor system are serious matters, and when they occur, they cause a fundamental deterioration in our lives. For thousands of years they have been associated with the disorders of aging and were therefore thought to be unavoidable and irreversible. But, as we shall see, they can be prevented and reversed.

Chapter 2

James (32 Years): The Nightmare Back

Chronic pain in the lower back is as American as apple pie. It is so common and so predictable that we are not surprised when it happens. But what physicians call the "lower back syndrome" is also as British as beef, as French as Brie, as German as beer, as Japanese as sake, and as Australian as Vegemite. Chronic lower back pains are so endemic to the industrialized nations that surveys in these countries suggest that up to three-quarters of the population over 45 suffer from them. The British physician Wilfred Barlow estimates that half of all the adult population of England suffers severe lower back pains and sciatica.[1]

There is a direct relationship between chronic back pain and stressful, challenging situations. It is even part of our modern folklore. To be a salesperson, to be a manager, to meet quotas, deadlines, and scheduled goals—all of which are basic procedures of modern business practices—is to risk incurring chronic back pain. We expect damage to occur to our bodies, even when we are not doing physical labor.

As it occurred to James. James was a technician in a television studio, a job he had held for more than 10 years. When he was in his mid-twenties, he noticed occasional twinges in his lower back, but they always went away. By the time he reached his late twenties, the pain was more common. He always had the same ache when he woke up, and it stayed with him until he began to be more active during the morning.

By the time he reached his early thirties, James's familiar morning ache had become chronic, a back pain that increased with a vengeance by late afternoon. He felt pain not only in the curve of his lower back but frequently down the back of his pelvis. It was hard for him to walk long distances. His stride was shorter, and he tired more easily. At the studio, his ability to lean forward and to reach the control panel had become both constricted and slower. If James worked in his garden on Saturday, he would be almost crippled Sunday morning. And on two occasions—once starting his lawn mower and again using a spade—his back suddenly "went out." Each time he froze with such intense pain that he had to stay in bed for a full week.

This was a nightmare for James, who otherwise was in perfectly good health, kept quite active, and had an athletic body. In fact, he used to jog regularly. At 32 he looked young and felt young, except that his body was "breaking down." Nothing seemed to help. If he rested and took painkillers, the pain would diminish, but it came back a few days later. The best remedy was a weekly visit to a chiropractor, which relieved the pain immediately. Within a day or so, though, the pain always returned.

James's doctor, after looking at X rays, said that his intervertebral disks were weakening and beginning to protrude as the posterior walls of the lumbar vertebrae narrowed—"disk degeneration," he called it. He showed James his X rays. They showed the lumbar vertebrae tilted backward in a swaybacked curve, with the posterior facets of the vertebrae looking as if they were falling into the disk material, which was protruding outward. The doctor said that if the disks became any weaker they might herniate or rupture, and then the only relief would be surgery, to remove the extruding disk material or to fuse the lower vertebrae. James's physician would not promise him one hundred percent recovery, only that surgery would avert paralysis.

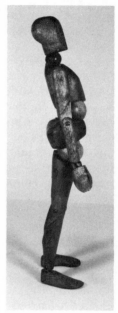

Figure 4
James's Posture

When I met James, he was in despair. But within two weeks he was no longer in pain; and he felt only a generalized stiffness which was rapidly disappearing, in his back and trunk. Within six weeks he had begun to jog again for the first time in five years.

What was wrong with James's back? Can a stressful job situation really cause disks to dissolve and bones to collapse? No, of course not. But long-term stress can cause an increasing contraction in the paravertebral muscles that run vertically down either side of the spine and attach to the upper portion of the sacrum. That's the origin of chronic stiffness and pain in the back.

When James told me his problem, I did two simple things: I touched him, and I looked at him. Palpation—feeling the patient's body—is almost a lost art in the medical world. Why touch patients if you can see inside their bodies with X rays? The reason is because X rays do not show the body's softer tissues, like the muscles. When I touched James's paravertebral muscles, I found that they were not soft, but rigidly contracted, almost like cables. And when I looked at him from the side, I saw that his lower back was curved into a swayback.

The swayback that I saw was precisely what the physician saw in the X-ray photo—the lower vertebrae tilted into an extreme lordotic curve, like an archer's bow. But, because the X rays did not show muscle contraction, they did not show the physician the taut thong that had pulled the bow into its curve. That thong was James's paravertebral muscles, chronically contracted, perhaps 50 percent, day and night. Research on extreme tonic muscular contraction has shown that it goes on uninterrupted even during sleep.[2] It is no wonder that James and others with this problem wake up sore.

The tremendous posterior tension of these hypercontracted paravertebral muscles had gradually curved James's vertebrae so that their rear surfaces were forced down into the disks, causing the disks to protrude slightly. The X rays gave the illusion of a stack of blocks collapsing from lack of support (Figure 5a). If we keep in mind, however, that this is not a structural pile of blocks but rather a musculo-skeletal system that is controlled by a brain operating in a stressful environment, we will see something quite different when we look at the X rays: a section of vertebrae that has been bowed under the stress of a chronically active muscular pull (Figure 5b). The root of James's back pain was sensory-motor amnesia, a problem that could be traced back to his brain.

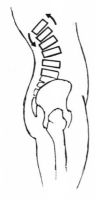

Figure 5a
"Collapsing Blocks" Illusion

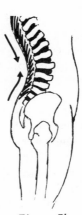

Figure 5b
Vertebrae Bowed by Muscular Pull

The moment we realize that James is a human with a brain, whose functions are however deficient, we know he can determine for himself what functional changes he needs to make. But if we think of James merely as a brainless mechanical doll with a collapsed spinal structure, then we have a desperate medical situation, one that demands a reengineering of the doll's spine—the operation James's doctor could not guarantee.

I treated James as a human being who could relearn to sense and control the hypertense muscles of his lower back. I had him lie down on a padded work table, to relieve his brain of its habitual response to having to support weight. I helped him feel movement in his pelvis and in the vertebrae of his lower spine. As he began to sense these movements, he informed me that he was becoming aware of that region of his back for the first time in years: "I'm beginning to feel what's there," he said. "Before, I didn't feel anything other than the pain."

Once this sensory feedback to the brain became clearer to him, I asked him to attempt gentle movements of the parts of his back he was beginning to perceive. We worked our way gradually along the full length of the spine, with James feeling and then lightly contracting the muscles that had automatically contracted up until this time. The paravertebral muscles slowly began to soften, and the extreme lordotic curvature began to release. I had him reach behind his back to feel the muscles, so that the sense of touch in his hands could add to his brain's internal sensing of his muscles' softening.

Once we had reestablished sufficient sensory-motor competence, I taught James a simple Somatic Exercise, one he could practice in the evening before bedtime and in the morning upon awakening. At these times, when the brain waves are slower, the brain is more open to new learning.[3]

James practiced these brief exercises in somatic control for a week. When he appeared for his second appointment smiling, I knew his sensory-motor amnesia was fading. He was out of acute pain now, and he could move more easily and with more confidence. We did some further exploration of spinal and trunk movements on the work table, and he learned a more ambitious Somatic Exercise. He went off for a second week of practice in relearning sensory-motor control.

When I saw him the next time, James reported that even the mild soreness he had felt was gone. Rather than complaining about pain, he now wanted his trunk to be even more supple. This meant to me that he had passed through the looking glass to the other side. He was no longer focused on how to get rid of pain, but on how to gain greater flexibility—signaling the rearrival of sensory-motor control. It was obvious to me that I was about to lose a client, and I congratulated James on this fact. For our third session we explored how greater control of the central muscles of the trunk now made possible greater freedom of movement of the shoulder and hip joints. I taught him a complex movement pattern involving the coordination of trunk, arms, and legs. Then I said good-bye to him as my client.

Years later I spoke to James and asked him how he was. He said he had no problems whatsoever. In the morning he still performed the Somatic Exercises I taught him. He didn't feel normal unless he reminded himself of how good it felt for his muscles to be long and relaxed. When he woke up, he "stretched like a cat" and then went to work. A couple of days a week he jogged in the early morning. The stress of television production was the same, but James wasn't the same. He was supple in his response to stress, and he enjoyed his work. "You were right," James said. "You can have your cake and eat it, too."

Interlude: **Chronic Muscular Tension**

James was fortunate in that we diagnosed and corrected his muscular tension early. He spent only a few years in pain. We could still have corrected his problem if he had come in later on in his life, but by then he would have undergone 20 or 30 years of pain. I have had many clients who experienced more or less constant pain in some part of their body for up to 40 years. They always had chronic muscular tension in these areas as well. Constant pain and chronic muscular tension go together. But they can be prevented from ever happening at all.

Muscles are designed for one action: to contract, or grow shorter. The contraction occurs when the muscle receives an electrochemical signal from the central nervous system to do so. When the signal stops, the contraction stops, and the muscle relaxes back to its former length. It does not take energy to relax and lengthen a muscle, only to contract and shorten it. When we voluntarily contract a muscle and then relax it, the muscle should soften almost completely. A relaxed muscle has absolutely no electrical activity in it. Full voluntary control of a muscle is the ability both to contract the entire span of the muscle and to relax it fully to its entire length.

Many people, however, contract the muscles of their backs or hips or shoulder in order to move. But then, when the movement is finished, they do not voluntarily relax the muscles back to their full length. Rather than the contraction and the energy consumption dropping down to zero, the muscles remain 10 percent contracted—or 20 percent or even 40 percent. No matter how hard they try, these people cannot fully relax their muscles. Their muscles continue to do work and to burn up energy.

All muscles have tone, or *tonus;* that is, a natural elasticity or ability to stretch and contract in response to stimuli. In the resting state, *tonus* is zero. So, if we have complete control of a muscle, we can achieve a *muscle tonicity* of zero—complete relaxation. But if we lose our voluntary control of the muscle, its tonicity can increase to 10, 20, or even 40 percent. This is chronic muscular tension.

If the tonus is 10 percent, the muscle will always feel tired and firm. If the tonus is 20 percent, the muscle will feel tired, very firm, and sore. If the tonus is 40 percent, the muscle will feel tired, hard, and quite painful. People with chronically high muscular tonicity often feel that their muscles are "weak" because they cannot move freely. Sometimes physicians will tell them that the muscles have become weak. On the contrary, their muscles are quite strong, but they are tired and overworked from contracting all the time. If we would only bother to feel our muscle, we would feel its hardness, a sure sign of its constant contraction. The chronically contracted muscle is like a motor that one cannot turn off. It continues to run and to burn up energy.

This is why muscles with a high tonus are always sore. The glycogen, which is stored in the muscle for the energy of contraction, is constantly being burned up. The combustion of glycogen creates contraction, and the glycogen is then turned into lactic acid. If there is constant combustion, then there is a constant buildup of lactic acid, and the more acid there is, the more the muscle's sensory cells become irritated. A constant 10 percent buildup will create enough activity to make the muscle feel tired. A constant 40 percent buildup will create so much hot acidity around the pain receptor cells that the bloodstream cannot flush it away, and the muscle will constantly feel painful.

It is common to have chronically sore or painful muscles from the late twenties onward. It can go on year after year, at times being hardly perceptible, but at other times intolerable, depending on how much stress the individual has endured. As we become older we have had time to accumulate many stressful and traumatic experiences. Therefore, in later years, we usually suffer greater muscular tonus, and thus more stiffness in our bodily movements, as well as a more distorted posture. Because of the constant production of lactic acid, these hard, stiff muscles are also chronically sore and painful.

This muscular stiffness, limitation of movement, tiredness, distortion of posture, and chronic pain are misinterpreted as the effects of "old age"—a fictitious disease that presumably leads to physiological degeneration, constant fatigue, and weakness and is "irreversible." In fact, however, age has nothing to do with it. These events are the result of an accumulation of physiological reactions to stress and traumatic accidents. Usually it takes a number of years to accumulate enough stress or trauma to raise muscle tonicity to such an unhealthy level. But the same chronic muscle tension can occur in a young person, if the childhood and teenage years were unusually traumatic. I have seen many people in their twenties and thirties with the same bodies, the same high tonicity, and the same complaints as those of people in their seventies. In every case they had suffered early childhood illnesses, surgery, a tragic family dislocation, or a threatening sociopolitical situation such as war.

Increasing muscular tonus usually occurs in later years. There is no question about that. But it occurs in later years, not because of the accumulation of the mysterious factor of "age," but because of the accumulation of the unmysterious factors of stressful living and traumatic accidents. The longer one lives, the more chances one has for these events to occur and accumulate. Some humans have an early and intense accumulation and so show these symptoms early. Others have the good fortune to escape these effects of stress or trauma, and they are just as supple and lively at 70 as they were at 25. It is my hope that, with increased understanding of sensory-motor amnesia, this latter group will grow in number.

When we consider that the human body has almost 800 muscles, and that all of them are well stocked with sensory cells, we can appreciate why our well-being depends on sensory information fed back to our brains by our muscles.

People with high muscle tonus do not feel good. Often they see no hope for recovery. "Oh, I feel so old!" hundreds of clients have told me, implying that their high degree of tonus is irreversible.

But muscular reactions to stress can be overcome. It is possible to feel genuinely "young" no matter what one's age. Practically speaking, this means to enjoy a muscular tonus that is very low in contraction and energy expenditure and very high in comfort and control. The basic somatic task during our lifetime is to gain greater and greater control over ourselves, learning to flow with the stress and trauma of life, like a cork floating on top of the waves.

Chapter 3

Louise (56 Years):
The Frozen Shoulder

When I met Louise, she had a "frozen shoulder." Two years earlier she had fallen, breaking the upper part of the humerus where the arm articulates with the shoulder. A surgeon had applied a pin to the bone to hold it together, and then removed it later on. The bone structure healed and was normal, but the arm functions did not heal. Physical therapy released some of the arm's post-surgical rigidity, but the improvement was minimal. Louise could not lift her right arm above the horizontal position, nor could she bring it behind her back. She could move her arm forward, but even this was difficult because she had intense chronic pain in the front of her shoulder joint. Louise, in her mid-fifties, had come to a decision: "I guess I'm just over the hill."

After Louise gave me her history, I had her stand up so that I could observe her stance and feel her muscles—just as I had done with Barney and James. Looking at her from the front, I could see that her right shoulder was lower than her left. It looked "pulled down," and her right hand hung three-quarters of an inch lower than her left hand. She said, "My arm feels like it weighs 50 pounds." She stood before me, looking despondent and wilted on one side.

When I touched her muscles, I immediately knew why her arm felt so heavy. She was correct: It was weighed down. There was a powerful contraction of the latissimus dorsi muscle, which attaches to the upper surface of the humerus and to the edge of the shoulder blade and then spreads down across the back to the lower spine and pelvis. This constant contraction pulled her arm down and prevented her from reaching above the horizontal level. In order to perform the simplest forward movements of her arm, like driving or eating, she was forced to exert an enormous contraction of the muscles on top of her shoulder. These muscles suffered intense chronic pain; they were constantly overworked. And the frozen latissimus dorsi muscle was out of her control.

Louise's powerful chest muscle, the pectoralis, was also involuntarily contracted and rigid. This muscle, next to the latissimus dorsi, has its roots on the upper surface of the humerus. Its fibers fan out in front of the chest, attaching to the clavicle, or collarbone, and sternum, or breastbone, and reaching all the

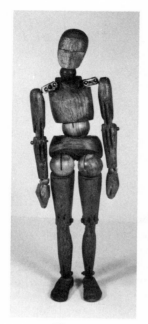

Figure 6
Louise's Posture

way down to the fifth, or sometimes the sixth rib. The rib cage, in turn, was pulled down by a chronic contraction of the abdominal muscle, which extends downward from the lower half of the chest to the pubic bone. The rigidity of the pectoral and abdominal contraction kept the shoulder held slightly forward and downward against the equally unremitting pull of the latissimus dorsi backward and downward. Thus, the shoulder was "frozen." It was as if Louise had a crippled wing.

Because Louise was in her fifties, she had assumed it was due to her age that her arm had not healed. Her physician told her that her arm was frozen by adhesions formed around the fracture that had occurred near the joint. He said that the adhesions might be removed by surgery. But, after two surgical interventions, setting the pin and removing it, Louise objected to further surgery. Curiously enough, she thought it would not help.

Louise was intuitively right: Surgery would not have helped her frozen shoulder, because it was not some "thing"—some structural blockage, such as "adhesions"—that prevented movement. Rather, regions of Louise's brain outside of her conscious control were continuously signaling for her muscles to contract. This distinction between a "thing" (i.e., a structure) and an ability (i.e., a function) is fundamental in viewing human problems somatically. If a "thing" is the cause, then some structure must be surgically cut or chemically altered. But if lack of voluntary ability is the cause, then a human function must be restored.

Specifically, Louise had to relearn to use her muscles efficiently, and that presented the problem. From my experience I knew what was causing her frozen shoulder, but all Louise could sense was a heavy right arm and an intense pain in the front of the shoulder. She was unaware of the contraction of her muscles. Not only could she not relax them, she could not even sense them. She believed, as her physician had told her, that some structure beyond her power to control was blocking her movement.

In order to restore Louise's voluntary ability to control the muscles that were "frozen," I had to help her become aware of the action of contraction from within her own central nervous system. While she lay on her left side, with a pillow under her head and her right side up, I placed one hand on her lower back at the borders of the latissimus dorsi muscle and the other on her right shoulder. I then moved them together so that she could perceive their connection.

Gradually she became aware that the movement in her lower back was directly connected with the movement in her shoulder. At that point, I asked her to do an odd thing: to contract the latissimus dorsi muscle as hard as she could all the way to the pelvis, making her shoulder even tighter and more "frozen." As she did this, I held her arm forward and pulled it firmly in the opposite direction, so as to make her contract even harder. Why did I make her do this? So that the sensory feedback would make her highly conscious that she was contracting her own shoulder into a frozen position.

Louise practiced voluntarily making her shoulder even tighter, alternately contracting, then releasing, the "frozen" muscle that had been spastically holding her arm. As she continued this movement, she got better at it: She was remembering how to do it. And the more she remembered, the better she became at it. Soon the release of the formerly spastic muscle was so successful that the muscle became soft and loose, allowing her shoulder to move freely for the first time in two years.

Louise was both exultant and amazed. She even began to weep at the magic of the transformation. And the joy of her tears was compounded by the expanding realization that she had regained control of herself. The magic was not in anything that I did; the transformation had occurred because Louise had accomplished it from within. She felt the expansive experience of rediscovering herself to be free and self-controlling.

We followed similar procedures with the other muscles of Louise's shoulder joint until both her sense of what she was doing and her motor control were sufficiently clear. I then taught her a Somatic Exercise that would let her rehearse her newly found sensory-motor ability just before going to bed and just after waking up. Two weeks later, in our third session, she lifted her right arm up to a vertical position and was able to put it against her right ear.

From that point onward Louise remained comfortable, supple, and active: Her shoulder problem did not return. And something else did not return: her despondent, "over-the-hill" feeling. She forgot that she was in her fifties and began acting like a much younger woman. The experience of discovering that she had within herself the resources to overcome a serious physical problem had given her vibrancy and confidence again.

Interlude: **What "Somatic" Means**

There are two ways in which a human being can be viewed: from the outside in, or from the inside out. Looked at from the outside, by a physiologist or a physician, human beings are very different from the beings they appear to be when they view themselves from the inside out.

When one looks at another human being, one sees a "body" with a certain external shape and size. It's just the same as an observed statue or wax dummy that also has a "bodily" shape and size. But when the human being looks at himself or herself from the inside, he or she is aware of feelings and movements and intentions—a quite different, fuller being. To view a body from the outside is a third-person view: One sees a "he" or a "she" or an "it." But when the human views himself or herself from the inside, it is a first-person view—a privileged view of "me," which means being aware of "I, myself."

What physiologists see from their externalized, third-person view is always a "body." What the individual sees from his or her internalized, first-person view is always a "soma." *Soma* is a Greek word that, from Hesiod onward, has meant "living body." This living, self-sensing, internalized perception of oneself is radically different from the externalized perception of what we call a "body," which could just as well be a human, a statue, a dummy, or a cadaver—from an objective viewpoint, all of these are "bodies."

Any viewpoint of the human being that fails to include both the first-person, somatic view and the third-person, physiological view is deceptive. To view a human only as a third-person, externalized body is to see only a physical puppet or dummy that can be changed by the external methods of chemical and surgical engineering. This is, *prima facie*, a false view of the human being: It is one-sided and incomplete.

Inasmuch as "scientific medicine" has built itself on the foundation of an objective, third person view of the human as a body, it is a deceptive and incomplete approach to human health. Scientific medicine not only ignores a fundamental truth about human beings but dooms itself to be consistently inefficient as a method of aiding human improvement. Because its view of the human being is insufficient, medicine's ability to help human beings is insufficient.

The uniqueness of human beings is in being, simultaneously, subjects and objects. Humans are self-sensing and self-moving subjects while, at the same time, they are observable and manipulable objects.

To yourself, you are a soma. To others, you are a body. Only you can perceive yourself as a soma—no one else can do so. But everyone else can see you as a body. Even you can see yourself as a body by looking into a mirror. In the mirror you will see an external, third-person "him" or "her" just like everyone else; but only you have the privileged perception of also seeing "me."

The great calamity of the human sciences is that we have, as it were, ganged up on ourselves. Only one person can see himself or herself as a first-person somatic being, but millions of people can see that person as a third-person bodily being. Consequently, these millions can join together and observe, measure, and diagram the objective body of the human person. That is the easy and obvious way taken by the sciences.

But what is easy and obvious is not necessarily true or effective. It is all very well for millions to study our objective bodies: There are some fundamental and essential facts to be ascertained about how humans are subject to the same physical and chemical forces as are all other bodies, from atoms to asteroids. But if these millions pursue their studies of human bodies as if humans were only third-person, objective bodies and not simultaneously first-person, subjective somas, then they are blind and dangerous. They are blind because they have trained themselves to see only one side of whole people: They ignore our somatic side. And they are dangerous, because their observations, predictions, and practical methods are based on a false, incomplete view of the human being.

The reason that physiology and medicine have failed to perceive the myths behind aging is that they have failed to recognize the fundamental fact that all human beings are self-aware, self-sensing, and self-moving: They are self-responsible somas. The somatic viewpoint recognizes not only that human beings are bodily beings who can become victims of physical and organic forces, but also that they are equally somatic beings who can change themselves. Humans can learn to perceive their internal functions and improve their control of their somatic functions.

This is the underlying theme of this book: that the somatic viewpoint must be added to the objective bodily viewpoint if we are to understand exactly what happens to human beings as they age. By adding the somatic viewpoint to our human sciences, we not only become capable of overcoming major health problems mistakenly attributed to aging, but we are capable of overcoming many of the major health problems that plague all of humankind.

In saying this, there is absolutely no implication that physiological science is invalid. On the contrary, its contributions to understanding the objective functions of the human being are monumental. What I am saying is that this contribution is, even so, incomplete and insufficient, and that this is clearly seen in the perennial incompleteness of medical diagnosis and the insufficiency of medical treatments in the areas I am discussing.

The somatic viewpoint complements and completes the scientific view of the human being, making it possible to have an authentic science that recognizes the whole human: the self-aware, self-responsible side as well as the externally observable "bodily" side. Together, these two viewpoints make possible an authentic human science. By completing a viewpoint of human beings that has, for so long, suffered from incompleteness, we will set foot on a new continent of human advancement.

Chapter 4

Harley (60 Years): The Retracted Landing Gear

Walking with a smooth, even stride is one of the essential human functions. We are bipedal creatures with a way of walking that is different from that of any other bipedal animal: Each arm swings freely to counterbalance the movement of the opposite leg. There is a twist in the middle of our spine, centering between the seventh and eighth rib vertebrae, at which point the upper body is rotating in one direction and the lower body in the other.[1]

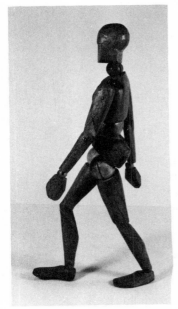

Figure 7a
Normal Bipedal Walking from Side

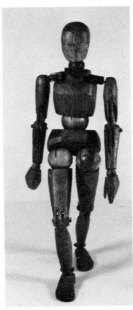

Figure 7b
Normal Bipedal Walking from Front

At least this is what happens in normal bipedal movement (see Figures 7a and 7b), which requires that the posture be vertical for these upper and lower rotations to be smooth and even. If the body's posture is bent or tilted, the smooth balance is utterly compromised, and one must walk with a slow, halting, uneven gait. When this happens, walking is inefficient, fatiguing, and often painful.

Harley walked into my office with a pronounced limp. His body lurched to the left, and he swung his left leg in an outward curve as he brought it forward. Otherwise, Harley was a hardy, ebullient man in his sixties with the look of a California rancher who had spent most of his life out of doors. A year or so earlier he fell out of a pickup truck and landed on his left knee, which became swollen and discolored and left him hobbled for a number of weeks. X-ray examination showed that, fortunately, the knee capsule was undamaged. The cartilage and tendons had been severely impacted and jerked, but they were intact. Even so, after the pain and swelling had faded away, Harley found that he walked with a stiffly bent left knee, his weight heavily pitched over onto the left leg. He had trouble just getting around, but what he missed most of all was square dancing with his wife.

I examined Harley's knee and found that it moved quite freely; and, when I manipulated the leg, it could straighten completely. There was no interior obstruction nor any grating sound, and there was no looseness in the capsule when I put lateral pressure on the knee joint. It was a perfectly sound knee, except that, while standing or walking, Harley could not straighten it. Already I knew that his problem was functional, not structural.

In standing, Harley tilted strongly to the left, with his head tilted back to the right in compensation. I asked him if the muscles on the right side of his neck were always sore, and he said yes. All the muscles on the left side of his trunk were rigidly tight, especially those in the left waist. These pulled his rib cage so far over to the left that it was touching his pelvis. It was as if these muscles were still cringing in response to the fall on his knee. In fact, this was precisely what was happening: The painful trauma of the fall had triggered in the brain a reflex muscular contraction on the left side, which had lingered on ever since the time of the fall. The shock to his left side—and to his right brain hemisphere—was, as it were, frozen in time.

The muscles of Harley's left waist and hip were so spastic that he could neither move nor straighten his leg in a normal fashion. His left pelvis and knee were

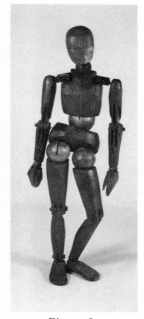

Figure 8
Harley's Posture

"frozen" in a bent, cringing position—like an airplane landing gear half re-tracted. Because medical technology allows doctors to focus only on the small picture, his doctors, in looking at the knee for structural damage, had missed the larger picture of what was actually happening to his entire left side.

I began to reacquaint Harley with the powerful muscles of his left side, which at that time he could not sense. The center of his sensory-motor amnesia was on the left of his body in the muscles attaching the rib cage to the pelvis. While he lay sideways on my work table, I moved his pelvis for him in the same way it would move if he voluntarily did it himself. As he began to sense movement in that part of his waist, I asked him to try to do it himself—voluntarily contract-ing the already tight waist muscles even a bit tighter.

Consider this from a functional viewpoint: Harley's waist muscles on his left side were constantly receiving a signal from the involuntary part of his brain to contract at, perhaps, 50 percent of their capacity. I asked him to contract them at 80 percent or more by sending an even stronger signal from the voluntary part of the brain. The electrochemical signal from the cerebral cortex, the vol-untary part of the brain, was stronger than the signal from the involuntary, subcortical portions of his brain. In electrochemical terms, the voluntary signal was "overriding" the involuntary signal and reasserting its control of the waist muscles. In this way, once Harley learned that he could voluntarily control his waist muscles, a magical event happened: They began to soften and lengthen for the first time in a year and a half.

Harley and I continued to practice this, until he became better at it. As he became better, not only did his ability to contract and release these muscles improve, but, equally, his sensing of this area of his body began to improve. As his hip relaxed down to its normal position, he was able to straighten his knee while walking.

"I feel like my left side is waking up again," Harley said. In fact, his brain was waking up; that is, the cerebral cortex, the seat of the brain's voluntary actions, had begun to take charge of his body again. It is a wonderful neurolog-ical fact that increasing bodily awareness means increasing neurological sensory awareness, and that this sensory awareness of the muscles goes hand in hand with voluntary motor control of the muscles. This is because the sensory-motor system is a "feedback loop": in other words, if you cannot sense it, you cannot move it, and the more you can move it, the more you will sense it. This is a rule of the sensory-motor system, one solid part of the neurophysiological founda-tion of somatic education.

I do not wish it to seem like I never spend more than three sessions with a client, but, as it turned out, Harley and I saw each other twice more and that was all. In the first session, I taught him control of his waist muscles; during the second, we focused on his hip muscles; and during the third we focused on coordinating his ankle and knee with his hip and waist muscles. At the end of the third session, Harley had no limp whatsoever. He walked with a smooth, even stride, his trunk vertical and his upper arms swinging freely in balance with the lower movements of his legs. Harley could straighten out his knee with total freedom, and he soon returned to his beloved weekly square dancing.

Interlude: **The Unconscious Levels of the Brain**

One of the most striking features about sensory-motor amnesia is that we are unconscious of muscle contraction while it is going on. It is a startling experience to discover that we are actively doing something without knowing it.

Every day I help my clients discover this aspect of SMA. For example, while a client with a chronically sore shoulder is lying on my padded work table, I lift her arm in the air and tell her to relax. Then, when I let go of her arm, it stays in the air. I call her attention to it: "Look at your arm. Do you notice something odd?" She looks and says, no, she sees nothing odd. "But you're holding your arm in the air!" "Oh!" she says, and abruptly drops her arm. "I didn't realize what I was doing." Or a person who constantly has a sore neck will be on the table, lying on his back, while I try to lift his head. I cannot lift it because the posterior muscles of the neck are rigid. I say to him, "Relax the muscles in the back of your neck so that I can lift your head." He voluntarily relaxes them, and I lift his head, then put it down. I wait two seconds and try again. It will not lift—the posterior muscles have become contracted again, but he is unaware of it. Without prompting, he is never aware of it. All day, every day, he tightly contracts the muscles in the back of his neck, totally unaware of them, and comes to me wondering why he has constant neck pain. The muscles are fatigued and sore from continually working—and he doesn't know he is doing it.

My clients have been told by other health professionals that there is some simple, underlying cause for their pain—a nerve is being pinched, there is a bone spur, there is bursitis, arthritis, tendinitis. In modern medicine, it sounds reasonable, so it seems equally reasonable to perform surgery around or to the pinched nerve, or to scrape the bone, or to inject various drugs into the area. When these remedies fail to relieve the constant pain, however, the patients are informed that they have permanent conditions and must learn to live with them.

Sustained muscular contraction will result in soreness or pain. Every athlete knows that, just like every soldier who completes his or her first 40-mile march. Whether it is voluntary or involuntary, sustained muscular contraction produces soreness. When SMA occurs in musculature, the involuntary contraction is sustained, not for one day—as with the athlete or soldier—but every day. It can continue unabated—and unnoticed—for weeks, months, years, or for an entire lifetime. It is common for SMA contractions in the lower back to occur in one's early twenties and continue unabated, with varying intensity, for the rest of a person's life.

I might say to my clients, "Look, can't you see that you're doing this to yourself? Stop contracting your muscles and the pain will go away!" I might say this. I might say it for an entire year, or for 10 years, but it would not make the slightest difference, except to drive them to despair. They cannot sense their muscular contraction through their ears, from me—they have to sense it inside their own bodies.

I have already discussed how our sensing and moving of muscles is a feedback loop, going from the muscle to the spinal cord and brain and then back again. This loop can also be a short route through the nervous system, going from the muscle into the spinal cord and back out again without involving the nerve routes up to the brain. This is the sensory-motor pathway taken when a physician taps her mallet just below her patient's patella, evoking the knee-jerk reflex. The sensory impulse of the tap goes to a specific segment of the spine and is relayed back with an automatic muscular contraction.

In SMA, the sensory-motor circuit becomes sidetracked from its usual route through the voluntary controls of the brain and then entangled in the reflex reactions of the brain's involuntary pathways. There is still the same sensory-motor feedback loop, muscle-to-brain-to-muscle, but, as the nerve impulses travel up the spinal column, they are, as it were, short-circuited: that is, the feedback of sensory-motor impulses takes place below the conscious level of the brain's voluntary functions.

This is not difficult to understand once we take into account the evolutionary layers of the human brain. Humans do not possess a single brain so much as they possess three brains working in coordination. Each level evolved out of the earlier level, and each layer has added refinements of function that were lacking in the operations of the earlier lower level. A breakdown in their coordination characterizes SMA.

Paul MacLean described this three-layer organization as the "triune brain."[2] The earliest layer, developed in primitive sea slugs and fish, controls essential functions like heart regulation, blood circulation, respiration, locomotion, and reproduction. Using the metaphor of a car, MacLean depicted this level as the "neural chassis." The next brain layer—according to MacLean's analogy—added "wheels" to the chassis. This intermediate level refined the essential functions of the first, organizing them into greater movement coordination, more organized attention to aggressive and defensive actions, and more concern for territoriality and social hierarchy ("pecking order"). In its full development, the intermediate level is the bearer of certain emotions: the fear that will make an animal withdraw, the anger that will mobilize an animal to attack, the sexual desire that will lead an animal to mating. These emotional functions show a higher sensitivity to surrounding conditions and what kinds of actions are appropriate responses. This level of brain function is powerfully present in the human brain and is a central source of involuntary, and thus unconscious, actions.

The highest level came with the emergence of the neocortex, which MacLean analogized to "the driver at the wheel of the neural chassis." This is the massive proliferation of gray cells in mammals, which developed further in primates, and which achieved its most complex development in the human species. The neocortex, an immense collection of nerve cells, is the seat of the voluntary learning and control that takes place in the rest of the brain. The source of conscious actions, this voluntary control center is a colossal organ of adaptation and learning. It possesses only primitive abilities at birth, but, as we mature, it gradually but steadily begins to learn all of the complex abilities and movements that we associate with growing up.

Maturation is the growth of greater and greater cortical learning. This process can continue indefinitely, improving and refining human actions, unless negative conditions force the brain into emergency actions in order to survive. Sustained stress and traumatic accidents are such negative conditions that sidetrack the voluntary cortex from its normal control of the sensory-motor system. When that occurs, the lower and more primitive regions of the first and second levels take control. It is a regression to involuntary reaction. This is what occurs with sensory-motor amnesia.

How much better it would be if we could always return control of our muscles to our voluntary cortex after moments of stress! Then the process of living would not be disrupted by the pain and disability associated with SMA. We would continue to mature throughout our lives, instead of expending our energy fighting, and involuntarily sustaining, needless muscular contractions. We would reach closer to our full potential as human beings. That is the hope of *Somatics*.

Chapter 5

Alexander (81 Years): *Los Viejitos*

The Tarascon region of southwestern Mexico is famous for its traditional *Danza de los Viejitos*—the "Dance of the Little Old Men." The little old men, wearing flat brim hats over long white beards, are all bent forward, leaning on their canes. They are garbed in the loose white shirts and pantaloons of the peasants of the land around the city of Patzcuaro.

Actually, inside these costumes of white hair and white garments are young boys with very fast feet. At the beginning of the music, the "little old men" stand motionless, looking not even capable of standing upright. Then, gradually, they begin to shift their bodies with the rhythm, their knees lift, their feet shuffle, and, before you know it, they are dancing a little quickstep movement that's dazzling in its rapidity. Then, just when you think they have reached their limit, the tempo of the music suddenly doubles to an incredible pace, and the little old men are dancing furiously, their legs and feet blurred as they drum out the rhythm upon the ground. During all of this, they never cease leaning forward onto their walking canes.

The citizens of Tarascon know the myth of aging and its image of the old man walking on "three legs." It shows a charming insight the way they present the notion that inside these *viejitos* are really young boys waiting for the sound of music to induce them to emerge once again into joyful dancing. What a wonderful transformation when an old body, seemingly incapable of youthful movement, suddenly shows such speed and flexibility!

Alexander was a man of 81 years who looked exactly like a *viejito*: He walked with a cane and was bent forward about 50 degrees from the vertical. His son brought Alexander to see me, informing me in ad-

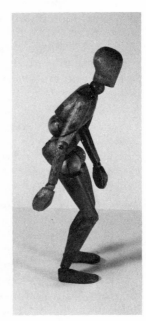

Figure 9
Alexander's Posture

vance that his father had constant pains in his chest and stomach. He was locked into his curvature of 50 degrees, so that when he slept on his back he had to have three large pillows under his head. This extreme posture is the very image of the old person in the riddle of the Sphinx.

Alexander's son told me that, given his father's age, he did not expect that anything could change his stooped posture, but he hoped I could relieve some of Alexander's chronic pains in the front of his body. Except for his posture, Alexander was a feisty, highly alert, person with no complaints except for the frequent ache in his stomach and lower back. His complexion was good, he ate well, he was interested in many activities, and he was, otherwise, quite healthy at 81.

His son said that Alexander's bending had begun in his mid-sixties, when he retired, and it had increased over a 15-year period. Once he got out of business, living on his investments and Social Security, Alexander apparently felt less in control of his economic destiny. He continually fretted over inflation and loss of stock values. It seemed that the more Alexander worried about his vulnerable economic position as a retiree, the more he doubled over.

As I do with all my clients, I looked at Alexander carefully from every angle while he was both standing and walking. I felt the muscles of his trunk to determine what was causing his postural distortion. His abdominal muscle was hard and leathery. The long abdominal muscle extends from the pubic bone and groin line all the way up to the center of the chest, covering over half of the front of the rib cage. When it is tight, it pulls the chest downward toward the pubic bone. When it is so tight as to be hard and leathery, it pulls the entire trunk forward into the typical curve of a *viejito*. The small intercostal muscles between Alexander's ribs were also excessively tight, depressing his chest wall, pulling his head forward, and distorting his neckline into a shape like that of a vulture.

As all athletes know, muscles that are used too much will be sore the next day. In Alexander's case, the muscles in his abdomen, chest, and neck were constantly in use and thus were constantly sore and fatigued. So were the muscles of his back, which were struggling to prevent his torso from completely collapsing. Because Alexander could not voluntarily release this contraction, he lived with constant pain and fatigue. He would wake up feeling full of energy, and then, within a couple of hours, he was dog-tired. Furthermore, the chronic contraction of his abdominal and chest muscles limited Alexander to very minimal, shallow breathing. His oxygen intake was not sufficient to metabolize his food, and that added to his constant fatigue.

Alexander's physician had explained to him that his feeling of weakness in the front of his body was due to atrophy of his muscles: They were supposedly degenerating. This, however, was the opposite of what was actually happening: Alexander's abdominal muscles were not weak at all, but incredibly powerful. They could not help but be powerful, because they were working constantly.

Realizing that Alexander's problems were due not to a degeneration of his bodily structure but to a dysfunction, I began to teach him how to overcome his essential difficulty: sensory-motor amnesia of the affected muscles. Because I didn't have three overstuffed pillows to allow him to lie on his back, I had him lie down on his side. With him in this side position, I did not attempt to straighten his trunk but did just the opposite: I made him more comfortable by curving him forward to almost 90 degrees. He liked that. I began to demonstrate what all his trunk muscles were doing while he was curled up. At first it was unclear to him what I was doing, but gradually he became aware of different areas in the front of his body.

I asked him to contract his abdominal muscles a little harder than they were already involuntarily contracted. At first he complained that he was too weak to do so, but gradually he began to achieve a moderate degree of voluntary contraction. As he did, he said, "I don't feel that pain in my stomach anymore."

We practiced in this fashion for a while, and then, to measure what changes he had made, I asked him to lie on his back. He protested, saying there would not be enough support for his upper trunk and head. I showed him a large pillow I had placed on the table. It was slanted up about 30 degrees from the surface. He said it was too low. I told him to try it and find out. He turned over and found that he could lie with his head against it. In less than an hour he had straightened 20 degrees!

I taught Alexander some Somatic Exercises to practice twice a day, at bedtime and upon awakening, and then sent him away. I didn't see him for a number of weeks, but I had reports from his son that the severe pains in his abdomen had disappeared, his sleeping was much improved, and he was considerably more energetic. He didn't become fatigued in the middle of the morning.

Six weeks later I saw Alexander for the second time, and during that session we gained further release in his abdominal muscles and began to do the same with the muscles of his neck. When, at the end, he lay down on his back, his head now came down to a 10-degree level. From that point on, he slept with only one pillow rather than three. His energy and range of activities improved enormously. The *viejito* had begun to hear his inner music again and had started to dance.

An even more significant change occurred in Alexander's life: He was less anxious. For years he had been cautious and crabby and fearful. Now, perhaps because he no longer felt constant pain, he was not as bothered by the things that used to trouble him. Consequently, he was clearer-headed in his thinking and decision making. His wife told me something more basic: He was much easier to live with—like he had been before he retired.

Alexander had been a captain of industry, with the power and perogatives of that position. Once he retired, he no longer felt the invulnerability that he had enjoyed throughout his working life. He had changed his entire life-style and modified the economic basis of his livelihood. Rather than being active in the affairs of the world, he was passive. Rather than being independent, he felt dependent on other forces. Retirement was a change that was very stressful for Alexander, and this continual stress had its somatic manifestation in abdominal muscular contractions. These contractions shortened his breath, pulled his trunk forward, and caused him to feel continual pain on top of his continual anxiety.

It was not old age that afflicted Alexander; it was growing sensory-motor amnesia in response to his radically changed life-style. It was not aging that caused the creature in the Sphinx's riddle to go from two legs to three; it was the same thing that had happened to Barney, James, Louise, and Harley—the negative effects of stress and traumatic injuries. When sensory-motor amnesia is avoided and the muscular response to stress and trauma are corrected, then "old age" disappears. There emerges from the little old men of Tarascon a concealed youth who begins to move in surprising ways.

Summary: **What These Five Case Histories Teach Us**

1. These problems are functional, not structural.   In all five case histories, the problems, which on the surface looked to be irreparable breakdowns of the body, were, instead, malfunctions of the nervous system. Viewed externally, they seem to be about five bodies that are degenerating; but viewed internally, these are five brains that have lost control of their bodily functions.

To use my own terms, these are somatic problems—not bodily problems. These are functional problems—not structural problems. These are problems solvable only by the patient—not by the doctor. These are problems reflecting a loss of control from the inside of the human system—not a deterioration of bodily parts at the outside of the human system.

2. The functional problems are cases of sensory-motor amnesia.   All five of these people were suffering from non-medical problems. They were outside the reach of medical help, whose services they had exhausted. They were not suffering from infectious diseases or physical lesions or biochemical imbalance. They were suffering from a loss of memory: the memory of what it feels like to move certain muscles of their bodies, and the memory of how to go about moving these same muscles.

Their memory loss was, to be specific, sensory-motor amnesia (SMA). I know this to be the case, simply because their being shown how certain muscular patterns feel, and how these contractions are accomplished, resulted in an end to their problems. They regained their normal functioning and normal bodily well-being without any need for antibiotics for infection or surgery for lesions or drugs to correct a biochemical imbalance.

3. These SMA problems were caused by the quality of their life span and not by the quantity: It was not the number of years but what happened during those years.   Age, in itself, is neutral as far as health is concerned. Age has never harmed anyone, nor has it ever killed a single human being. It is what happens during the aging process that harms and kills human beings.

Everything that happens to us during our lives causes a necessary reaction in our central nervous system. Our brain responds to and adapts to the events that occur. If we live a restricted, narrow life, our brain adapts to it. If we suffer years of anxiety, fear, and despair, our brain adapts to it. If we suffer shocks, accidental injury, serious illnesses, or complex surgery, our brain responds and adapts to it. These are the events that bring on sensory-motor amnesia, causing us to believe we are helplessly deteriorating. On the other hand, if we enjoy years of contentment, confidence, and hope, our brain adapts to that. And with very different effects.

The brain is an adaptive organ. It responds to the events of our lives in whatever way is necessary in order to survive and keep going. But, because the brain directly or indirectly controls all of our bodily functions, this means that our entire body reflects what has happened to us during our lifetimes.

The bodily malfunctions in all five of these case histories clearly reflect an internal, somatic adaptation to specific events that had occurred during the course of these lives. SMA is the unfortunate result of specific adaptations made by the central nervous system in response to what happens to us during our lifetimes. Part 2 is a discussion of these specific adaptations.

4. SMA always affects the entire somatic system and has its roots in the center of the human body.   Any imbalance in the sensory-motor system creates imbalance throughout the entire body. When the muscles in one single limb become spastic or clumsy or too flaccid, this loss of control and efficient coordination within the musculoskeletal system causes an automatic compensation within all the other interconnected bodily parts. The brain brings about these compensations automatically and unconsciously, in an attempt to rebalance the entire system.

Obviously, this compensatory rebalancing causes a distortion of the somatic functions internally and the bodily structure externally. The entire somatic system malfunctions and becomes askew. Because it is genetically programmed to preserve the somatic system, the brain rebalances and compensates for this imbalance, but the whole system has now become inefficient, less supple, slower in response, habitually self-stressed, and operating with a significant loss of energy. These are precisely the symptoms of what we mistake for "old age."

But not only does SMA always affect the entire somatic system, it also has its roots in the center of the human body: namely, in the waist, lower back, and abdomen where massive, powerful muscles connect the vertebrae and rib cage to the pelvis. This area is the center of gravity for the human body. And it is precisely the area where symptoms of "old age" first begin.

In sum, because any sensory-motor disturbance will affect not only the entire somatic system but also, and particularly, the gravitational center of the human body, two simultaneous, interconnected problems will occur. First of all, malfunctions will occur in the muscles at the center of gravity, which will cause malfunctions in the movements of (1) the spinal-pelvic centrum; (2) the shoulder and hip joints; (3) the elbows and knees; and (4) the distal regions of wrists and hands and ankles and feet. Conversely, the other problem is that injuries and malfunctions in the distal regions of the wrists and hands, ankles and feet, elbows and knees, shoulder and hip joints, and spine will cause malfunctions in the proximal muscles at the spinal-pelvic center of gravity.

This phenomenon was clearly present in the five case histories. In all five, the muscles in the center of the body are crucially involved, no matter what the specific problem was in the peripheral parts of the body.

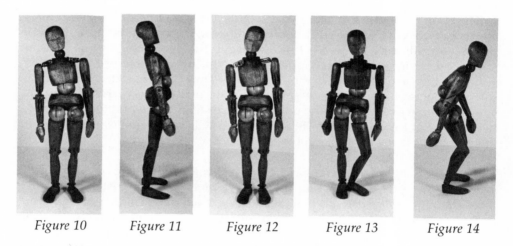

Figure 10   *Figure 11*   *Figure 12*   *Figure 13*   *Figure 14*

The specific problem with Barney's hip was that the muscles on the right side of his back were involuntarily contracted: The entire right rib cage was pulled down toward the side of the pelvis, causing his scoliotic leaning and distorted sense of balance (see Figure 10).

The specific problem with James's back was that the massive paravertebral muscles connecting the lower spine and rib cage to the pelvis were involuntarily contracted: The entire lower rib cage was pulled down into a bowlike curve toward the back of the pelvis, inhibiting both his walking and his reaching movements (see Figure 11).

The specific problem with Louise's shoulder was that the muscles of the shoulder girdle reaching downward on the right side of the trunk were involuntarily contracted: The entire shoulder-arm joint was pulled down, front and back, toward the pelvis in a "frozen" position (see Figure 12).

The specific problem with Harley's limping gait and bent knee was that the muscles of his left waist were involuntarily retracted upward to their attachments on the left rib cage and spine: The entire hip and leg were held upward like the half-retracted landing gear of an airplane (see Figure 13).

The specific problem with Alexander's stooped posture was that the abdominal muscles connecting the chest to the pubic bone and lower pelvis were involuntarily contracted: His entire trunk was pulled forward and downward into the classic stoop of senility (see Figure 14).

But, in all five, the basic problem was really the same: involuntary contraction of the muscles in the body's center of gravity, affecting the periphery of the body; or involuntary contraction in the periphery of the body, causing a compensating contraction in the center of gravity. In all five cases, the powerful muscles connecting the spine and rib cage to the pelvis were the root of the specific problem of each person.

Barney's hip, James's back, Louise's shoulder, Harley's limp, and Alexander's stoop were different manifestations of the very same event: chronic muscle contractions in the center of the body, which they could neither sense nor control, that were directly connected with chronic contractions in the periphery of the body.

Finally, it should be remembered that, in all five case histories, it was by becoming conscious of feelings and voluntary movements in the center of their bodies that these persons overcame the unconscious and automatic reflex contractions that the SMA had caused.

5. *Viewed internally and functionally, SMA is a single somatic problem. Viewed externally and structurally, SMA is a multitude of mysterious medical problems.* As I pointed out earlier, age is not the cause of anything, healthy or unhealthy. "Age" is a neutral term, just like "life": To live is to age. Nonetheless, within the medical profession and in medical research, the word age has a mysterious meaning. Even though, by definition, the word has no pathological significance at all, in medical usage, it has strong pathological significance: It is the mysterious unknown cause of all the mysterious symptoms in elderly humans that one cannot effectively diagnose or treat. "Doctor, why can't I be helped?" "Well, you're not getting any younger. After awhile things begin to break down. It's more or less what you should expect at your age."

This, of course, is nonsense. Age has nothing to do with the hundreds of problems it is blamed for. "Age" is a crypto-pathology. Behind the mystery lies ignorance, which is, by and large, an ignorance of the somatic condition of sensory-motor amnesia.

The five case histories are the prototypes of millions of case histories and of typical symptoms that occur all over the globe every day. Over a 12-year period, I made note of some of the complaints my clients had when they first came to see me. All of them had a clear connection with the central muscles of the body, and all were resolved when these muscles no longer constrained the other body areas they affected. In every instance, SMA was the single, somatic problem at the root of the multitude of mysterious symptoms.

In addition to painful feet, toes, legs, buttocks, chests, arms, hands, backs, necks, and jaws, my clients reported such symptoms as sciatic pains in the leg, swollen knees, varicose veins, weak ankles that turned too easily, stiff ankles that would not turn, leg cramps, numbness or "pins and needles" in their hands, chronic tension headaches, ringing in the ears, eye aches, shallow breathing, constipation, frequent urination, spasms of the urethra, inflamed joints, and restricted movement of the head. All of their complaints were chronic, all of them unresponsive to medical and paramedical treatments, and all of them resolved once the SMA was cleared up.

Please note that I do not say that all of them were "cured." Curing is a medical procedure which has no significance in respect to SMA. Curing and treating are what is done to a passive patient—an external engineering feat that goes from the outside to the inside. Sensory-motor remembering is an educational procedure, done by an active person—an internal somatic feat that goes from inside the brain to the muscle system.

All of the complaints mentioned above were what my clients felt and described. It was not what their physicians and other health professionals described. They had been diagnosed by medical specialists as having neuralgia, scoliosis, kyphosis, lordosis, arthritis, bursitis, osteoarthritis, osteoporosis, spinal stenosis, bone spurs, carpal tunnel syndrome, compressed disks, bulging disks, slipped disks, herniated disks, degenerated disks, subluxated disks, hypochondria, allergic reactions, postsurgical trauma, and, in the end, "undiagnosable pain."

From the medical viewpoint, the fact that the complaints, so diagnosed, persisted despite medical treatment meant that they were "incurable" and therefore the fault of old age. But, from the somatic viewpoint, this was only part one of a two-part investigation, the second of which disclosed that sensory-motor amnesia—particularly of the muscles of the body's center of gravity—was the cause of these functional problems. Such functional problems cannot be "cured" by "treatment"; but they can be controlled, by relearning. Fortunately, that is just what happened to thousands of people with the complaints and diagnoses listed above.

PART 2

How Sensory-Motor
Amnesia Occurs

Chapter 6

Atrophy: The Role of Gradual Surrender

No advice is more treacherous than this: "Now that you're getting older, you ought to slow down a bit." This is a pathway leading directly to decrepitude. Such advice is not only debilitating; it is also deadly.

It is part of the traditional myth of aging that increasing age should mean decreasing physical activity. But folk wisdom can be profoundly wrong. In this case, it helps bring on the very loss of well-being that it presumes to avoid.

The truth is very different. If you want to pin a motto on your wall, pin up this one: "Function maintains structure." The more popular motto is, "Use it or lose it." This advice is correct, anatomically, physiologically, and neurologically. For example, if our bones are not regularly used to bear substantial weights and to sustain strong forces, they become soft. If our muscles are not regularly used in challenging and skilled activities, they become weaker and less responsive. If our brain cells are not systematically involved in a wide variety of voluntary activities, they deteriorate.

This softening, weakening, and deterioration of our resources takes place gradually and insidiously—not because of aging but because of what we cease to do as we age.

Those who believe that they should take it easy as they become older are deluded; they are persons who are surrendering their life functions bit by bit. For most people, the act of growing up, maturing, and settling down to adult life is an act of decay. It is a deliberate, and usually well-calculated, act of gradually giving up the functional abilities acquired during the process of growing up.

Maturation is a long process of learning, during which a repertoire of functions is built up which allows us to live life fully. But this is not what usually happens. No sooner do we acquire our repertoire of useful functions than we cease to use them—an instance of planned obsolescence. It is ironic that so many people complain about the breakdown of their refrigerators and automobiles, blaming the manufacturers for deliberately built in attrition of their products, yet often have bodies that are breaking down from the deliberate attrition that is built into their way of life.

Indeed, it is part of the American Dream to "have it made," it being clearly understood that a person who "has it made" is a person who has attained the status of doing nothing—of being inactive. A body in a bathing suit by a swimming pool, lying motionless on a chaise lounge, is the American image of "having it made." We should not forget, however, that this is also the image of a dead body.

To become an adult means that we no longer have to do the things we did as kids. Kids run, but we adults walk. Kids climb, but we take the elevator. Kids scoot under bushes, but we go around them. Kids stand on their heads, but we sit on our bottoms. Kids roll on the ground, but we turn on the mattress. Kids jump up and down, but we shrug our shoulders up and down. Kids laugh with joy, but we smile with restraint. Kids are exuberant, but we are careful. Kids want to have fun, but we want to have security.

In short, to become a successful adult means to cease acting like a kid. It is the customary sign of adulthood to cease functioning like a young person. But this conception of adulthood has an unavoidable result: As soon as we stop using these functions, we lose them. And we lose them because our brain, which is a highly responsive organ of adaptation, adjusts to this lack of activity. If certain actions are no longer part of our behavioral inventory, our brain crosses them off. In a word, it forgets. The practical, everyday awareness of how these actions feel and how they are performed fades away, and SMA is the result.

Physiological and Anatomical Research on Aging and Physical Activity

We now know it to be a fact that, as one becomes older, physical activity becomes more necessary, not less. In a 10-year study of 268 people over the age of 60, Palmore reported that degree and frequency of illness was related more directly to physical inactivity than to such well-publicized factors as smoking and being overweight.[1] Those who were physically inactive were two-and-a-half times more likely to spend at least 14 days a year bed-ridden as were those who were physically active!

During this same 10-year longitudinal study, Palmore discovered something of equal importance: The physically inactive were four times more apt to rate their health as poor as were those who were active. Worse, these indolent elders were twice as likely to report failing health when they appeared for their regular medical examination. Worse still, over 50 percent of these same inactive persons died sooner than actuarily expected, compared to between a fourth and a third of those who had more locomotor activities. Thus, as we reduce our sphere of physical activities, we reduce our chances for health and longevity.

Other research studies are more specific on the effects of regular physical activities. In Los Angeles at the Andrus Gerontology Center, DeVries reported that a well-planned program of physical conditioning leads to improvement in cardiovascular functioning.[2] The heart functions better, the blood pressure load is reduced, nervous tension decreases, further normalizing blood pressure, and the percentage of body fat drops, reducing the statistical probability of heart attack.

The *Journal of Gerontology* reported on the physiological effects of a month-long program of endurance training conducted with a group whose average age was 70.[3] Results: Reduction in circulatory stress, as evidenced by decreases in work pulse, in systolic blood pressure after exercise, and in blood lactate concentration. Barry, Steinmetz, Page, and Rodahl, and others, who carried out this experiment, found, at its conclusion, that the work load limit of these 70-year-old citizens was 76 percent higher than it was a month before! Additionally, the subjects showed improved oxygen uptake and pulmonary ventilation, as well as improvement in their postexercise systolic blood pressure and blood lactate level. Similar findings have been reported in many other studies published in the *Journal of Gerontology,* the *Journal of the American Geriatrics Society,* and others.

The British researcher, E. J. Bassey, states flatly that, "It is clear that training can improve the physical condition and maximum capacities of the elderly. . . ." He goes on to say that a physical training program, by itself, ". . . will bring no lasting benefit unless it catalyses a change to a more active life style which incorporates an appropriate amount of spontaneous exercise."[4] This, of course, means a more active life-style than that usually chosen by adults in their middle years, especially following the crucial time of their retirement.

There has been, in addition to American and British research, a significant amount of Soviet research into the effects of exercise on older persons. Soviet scientists have found that the human organism remains highly functional and adaptive as long as it is given suitable challenges to which it can respond.[5] When this occurs, there are positive effects on the adrenals, blood chemistry, carbohydrate metabolism, the cardiovascular system, the respiratory system, and the nervous system.

On an anatomical level, Smith and Reddan's studies in a female nursing home[6] have shown that regular physical exercises slowed bone loss and promoted bone accretion. This is a significant finding, inasmuch as fear of fractures, especially of the hip, normally motivates elderly females to become cautious in their locomotor activities. Just the reverse is their best protection.

In a similar vein, Erickson has studied the relation of joint flexibility to physical activity. He found that the collagen meshwork in the connective tissues shortens if it is not regularly stretched.[7] Again, maintaining a broad range of physical activity prevents joint stiffness and, hence, limited movement. In sum, and quite apart from SMA, both the function and the structure of the human body decline unless physical activity is constantly maintained.

Neurological Research on Aging and the Brain

As the riddle of the Sphinx makes clear, it is the loss of control of physical movement that inspired the myth of aging. During our middle years, we usually observe the start of impaired motor performance, including slower movement, decreased strength, and a loss of fine motor coordination.

For almost a century this has been explained scientifically as neurological. In the 1890s, Hodge, a neurologist, performed neuron counts on the brains of young and old humans. His conclusion was: "As the work of life is being done, the cells, one by one, are worn out. A stage is reached when only enough cells remain to barely support processes requisite for life. . . ."

This happens not to be true; but, unfortunately, later research did not correct this widespread misunderstanding. One still finds statements, in college text-books as well as in popular publications, to the effect that, soon after infancy, the brain begins to lose its fixed supply of neurons and that this loss continues until the end of life. Such information reinforces the myth of aging and leads us to the melancholy conviction that each day of our lives thousands of brain cells are flowing out of our heads as we steadily lose both our mental and our physical competence.

Eventually it was discovered that the task of counting the estimated 100 billion neurons of the brain demands a much greater scientific sophistication than that which was available to Hodge during the 1890s. The task is so complicated that even the most advanced microscopic and computer technology cannot solve the puzzle.

The Aging Motor System summarizes the full body of research done on aging and the brain. In it, the question of research reports on neuron loss is addressed head on: "The generalization to be gleaned from this body of reports is that at present there is no generalization about neuron loss in old age."[8]

Spelled out more fully by researchers Curcio, Buell, and Coleman, this means that

> As objective quantitative data accumulate at an increasingly rapid pace, it is becoming clear that age-associated declines are not universal or inevitable. Some aspects of performance do not decline; neuron loss with age is not found in all regions of the nervous system; not all neurons atrophy; not all transmitter systems decline; some neurological measures do not show decrements; and some degree of neuronal plasticity is retained in the aged nervous system.[9]

This statement adds credence to my own point of view.

In this same volume, Lars Larsson reviews the subject of "Aging in Mammalian Skeletal Muscle." He delineates three levels that should be examined for the effects of aging on muscular function: the brain, the motoneurons that conduct nerve impulses from brain to muscle, and the muscle itself. To account for the motor impairment that afflicts so many elderly persons, he concludes that "the factors of greatest importance appear to be reduced nerve impulse activity related to progressive disuse together with functional impairment and subsequent loss of motoneurones."[10] What he is saying is that reduced nerve impulses from the brain, along with an increasing disuse of muscles, results in impairment of muscle function as well as of the motoneurons immediately involved. The problem originates, thus, in an inability of the brain to send nerve impulses.

Larsson is referring in general to what I describe specifically as the condition of sensory-motor amnesia.

Fortunately, SMA can be corrected. The three editors of *The Aging Motor System* see three ways to prevent and treat this functional loss: by drugs, by behavioral retraining, and by preservation of physical fitness. They see some possibilities in drug treatment that need to be explored. They also see some behavioral training techniques as a way to relearn motor skills; but they conclude that, "finally, the maintenance of physical fitness through a life-style of daily exercises may offer an inexpensive and safe method to prevent motor and mental performance deterioration."[11]

In sum, the best of our scientific knowledge points directly to what I am suggesting in this book: that many of the physical problems attributed to old age are instead functional problems of disuse. I describe this as sensory-motor amnesia, the effects of which are temporary and can be prevented, or corrected, by means of a neurologically based exercise program such as the Somatic Exercises I present in Part 3.

Chapter 7

The Muscular Reflexes
of Stress

Hans Selye is one of the prime figures in twentieth century medical research. It was Selye's decades of work in endocrinology that led to his formulation of the concept of stress, and to a recognition of the fact that there are "diseases of adaptation."

Selye's formulation of the general adaptation syndrome (GAS) is, possibly, the most significant single event in medicine since the discovery of the germ theory of disease and the development of antibacterial drugs. The extraordinary significance of Selye's research is that it introduced into medicine what we have termed a "somatic" dimension: namely, the viewpoint that psychological events are as important as physiological events in determining human health or illness. The somatic viewpoint encompasses how we individually view ourselves from the inside looking out and how, from that viewpoint, the distinction between mind and body disappears. From inside ourselves, we are not aware of the "body" itself but rather of the feelings and active processes of that "body."

Hans Selye's somatic viewpoint has expanded the dimensions of health research by emphasizing the health importance of what we, from the inside of ourselves, can do to reduce the effects of stress by our own attitudes and by the way we control our lives.[1] This emphasis on self-responsiblity is a hallmark of the somatic viewpoint.

Traditional medicine emphasizes the external viewpoint of what can be done *to* the individual's body to improve health. Selye, while fully accepting this emphasis, expanded the dimensions of medicine to include the individual's internal ability of self-control. The somatic viewpoint does not subtract from medicine; it adds to it a recognition of the mind–body interaction that is involved in all diseases of adaptation. Here is the way Selye expresses it:

> Life is largely a process of adaptation to circumstances in which we exist. A perennial give-and-take has been going on between living matter and its inanimate surroundings, between one living being and another, ever since the dawn of life in the prehistoric oceans. The secret of health and happiness lies in successful adjustment to the ever-changing conditions on this globe; the penalties for failure in this great process of adaptation are disease and unhappiness.[2]

But , in addition to this general evolution of life,

> . . . there is another type of evolution which takes place in every person during his
> own lifetime from birth to death: this is adaptation to the stresses and strains of
> everyday existence. Through the constant interplay between his mental and bodily
> reactions, man has it in his power to influence this second type of evolution to a
> considerable extent, especially if he understands its mechanism and has enough
> will power to act according to the dictates of human intellect.[3]

Selye's viewpoint admirably expresses my own perspective. In fact, his definition of stress is essential in understanding the theme of this book: "In its medical
sense, stress is essentially the rate of wear and tear in the body." Stress, in itself,
is neither good nor bad; it is "the nonspecific response of the body to any demand."[4] To live means that we have continuous demands made on our bodies;
thus, how we respond and adapt to these ongoing demands will determine how
well our bodies stand up to the demands of living.

But, you will notice, to talk about stress is simply to talk about the nature of
living—of how well we cope with the daily demands placed upon us. This
means that stress is part of the nature of aging: How well we respond to it
determines how we age. Selye is addressing the same general question we have
been discussing all along. Indeed, by rephrasing what we have presented up to
this point, we can say that, "In its medical sense, what we have traditionally
taken to be the effects of aging is essentially the rate of wear and tear in the
body." The so-called "diseases of aging" are, as we have maintained, largely
"diseases of adaptation." Moreover, we have the power to influence this rate of
wear and tear if we have "enough will power to act according to the dictates of
human intellect."

The research of Hans Selye succeeded in expanding the dimensions of medicine by showing the effects that stress can have on the endocrine system when
it adaptively responds to some demand placed upon the whole bodily system.
In his general adaptation syndrome, he describes this response as having three
stages: the alarm reaction, the stage of resistance, and the stage of exhaustion.

Almost any event can cause an alarm reaction—anything from running a mile
to going without sleep, to having a violent argument, or to visually adjusting
from the dim light of a movie house to the bright sunlight outdoors. The demand placed upon the system brings about a protective adjustment; for example, the stimulation of the adrenal gland: Its secretion of epinephrine and
norepinephrine wakes up and mobilizes the biological resources of the body to
resist the stressor. Usually, this is the limit of the stress reaction. But, if the
period of resistance goes on for too long a time, increasingly depleting the
body's resources for resistance, a stage will be reached when these resources are
exhausted. Then a genuine breakdown can occur.

The GAS is an unavoidable and normal process that has been documented
by Selye in some 30 books. Selye's research centered primarily on the glandular

system, referring only generally to the effects of stress on the neuromuscular system. He recognized that, when we are under stress, increased muscular tension is inevitable, and suggested various attitudes and relaxation practices that can help to reduce it. But his research did not specify just what neuromuscular events occur with stress.

During the 12 years of my practice as a somatic educator, I have had ample opportunity to observe the specific effects of stress on the neuromuscular system. My findings, which I present in the next two chapters, help to round out Selye's initial discoveries regarding the stress response—specifically, the biochemical side of stress. By looking at the stress response more closely, we shall discover that it has a sensory-motor side as well, that is of equal importance to the biochemical side explored by Selye.

What I have found is that the neuromuscular system has two basic responses to stress, both of which have their focus in the middle of the human body, at its center of gravity. These two basic responses differ from one another because they are two very different forms of stress—what Selye would distinguish as "distress" and "eustress."

The neuromuscular adaptation to sustained negative stress ("distress") is the withdrawal response, which occurs primarily in the front of the body. The neuromuscular adaptation to sustained positive stress ("eustress") is the action response, which occurs in the back of the body. It is easier to think of the withdrawal response as the Red Light reflex. The action response may be thought of as the Green Light reflex. I discuss the Red Light reflex in the following chapter. The Green Light reflex is the subject of Chapter 9, and the trauma reflex, which is somewhat different, is discussed in Chapter 11.

Chapter 8

The Red Light Reflex

The Abdominal Muscles and the Withdrawal Response

It is surprising that a single, lower-brain reflex could be the cause of so many of the body changes that are associated with aging. It is also enlightening, because it helps us toward both understanding and overcoming the myth of aging.

"What with raising three children and taking care of the house and my husband, it's no wonder I have these crow's feet next to my eyes"—so says a wife. "If you want to know what it's like, keeping up a house, a wife, and raising three children, just look at the wrinkles on my brow. That's what worry will do to you"—so says a husband. Both husband and wife give witness to the same ancient reflex.

"I'm beginning to get a bump on the back of my neck, just like my aunt. Is that what they call a dowager's hump? And my head: It's always hanging forward. It looks just awful, like an old person's. Can you do anything about that?" This is a manifestation of the same lower-brain reflex.

"I sure wish you could do something about my shoulders. My wife says they slump. I used to have a fairly big chest, and now you can hardly see it anymore, its gotten so flat." The effects of the withdrawal response over the years did this.

"You know, I'm not even 60 yet, and already I stand stooped forward. The other day I saw this reflection in a store window of an old man bent over like he needed a cane. Then I realized it was me!" What he saw was a reflection of the Red Light reflex.

"My problem is that I can't get my breath anymore. I used to be able to climb the steps up to my front door and not think a thing about it. Now I have to stop to catch my breath. What's happening to me? Are my lungs beginning to shrink?" Again, this is the same reflex, so often evoked and so familiar that it becomes an unconscious habit. Only its effects are noticed.

"I've been active all my life, and I used to be able to outwalk anybody. But something's gone wrong with my thighs: They're sore all the time. And my knees, too. They ache when I get up in the morning." These, too, are effects of the withdrawal reflex.

For many decades neurobiologists have been fascinated with this human reflex, because it occurs throughout the entire animal kingdom. It is sometimes referred to as the "startle response"; at other times it is referred to as the "escape response," because it aids the animal in avoiding or evading a threat. It is a primitive reflex of survival. Its action in the central nervous system is usually mediated by "giant" nerve fibers large enough to allow the nerve impulse to travel more quickly. It is a "rapid motor act" that is built into the circuitry of even very simple organisms, helping them to survive by rapidly withdrawing from danger.

When you touch a sea anemone, its circle of small tentacles quickly retracts, drawing back from the threatening stimulus. A common earthworm exhibits an immediate withdrawal response when its body is touched by a probe. The pesky but clever fly will wait until you have just about reached it before abruptly withdraws, evading your fly-swatter. Its threshold for danger is high. Fish respond with fast get-aways, and crayfish with a sudden tail-flip response.

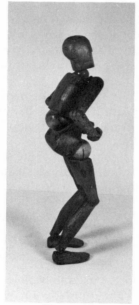

Figure 15a
Withdrawal Response: Side View

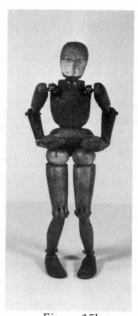

Figure 15b
Withdrawal Response: Frontal View

All mammals that have been studied exhibit the withdrawal response (see Figures 15a and 15b). Even in these complex animals, the reflex is quick and effective. And in the most complex mammal, the human being, the withdrawal response is amazingly quick. If a woman walking down a street hears the sudden explosion of a car backfiring, this is what happens: Within 14 milliseconds the muscles of her jaw begin to contract; this is immediately followed about 20 milliseconds later by a contraction of her eyes and brow. But, before her eyes have squeezed shut, her shoulder and neck muscles (the trapezius) have received a neural impulse at 25 milliseconds to contract, raising her shoulders and bringing her head forward. At 60 milliseconds, her elbows bend, and then her hands begin to turn palms-downward. These descending neural impulses continue by contracting the abdominal muscle, which brings her trunk forward, simultaneously pulling down her rib cage and stopping her breathing. And, immediately after that, her knees bend and point inward, while her ankles roll her feet inward. The muscles of the crotch tighten, and the toes lift upward. This sums up the Red Light reflex—the body's withdrawal from danger. The body is flexed and crouched, almost as if ready to fall and curl up in a fetal posture.[1]

This cascade of neural impulses begins in the face, then goes down to the neck, then to the arms and trunk, and, finally, to the legs and toes. Why this sequence from the head downward? Because the impulse originates in the lower-level brain stem and arrives at the muscles of the head region earliest, taking time to travel down its nerve pathways to the lower parts of the body.

This withdrawal response, shared by humans with the rest of the animal kingdom, emanates from the primitive regions of the hindbrain—to be precise, from the reticulospinal tract originating from the ventral pontine and medullar reticular formation.[2] Thus, the mechanism of this reflex lies deep beneath the control of the forebrain where conscious, voluntary actions originate. Not only is the withdrawal reflex more primitive than our voluntary actions, it is much faster. It happens before we can consciously perceive it or inhibit it. It is our primitive protector, whose motto is "Withdraw now, and think about it later." Survival demands an immediate response. We do not have the luxury to reflect at length on how dangerous the sudden threat really is.

As the Red Light reflex rapidly courses downward from head to legs, it causes contractions in exactly the same areas that I mentioned in the beginning of the chapter: the crow's feet and wrinkled brow, the dowager's hump and projected head, the slumping shoulders and flat chest, the stooped trunk, the lack of breath, and the aching knees. Because all of these are body changes associated with aging, it is surprising that they could be caused by a single, lower-brain reflex.

By recognizing the known and well-researched effects of the withdrawal response, we can gain simultaneous insight into two matters of great importance: (1) the specific responses made by our neuromuscular system to stress conditions; and (2) the real cause of body changes that, traditionally, and mistakenly have always been blamed on a fictitious disease called "aging."

Malfunctions Caused by the Withdrawal Response

The Red Light reflex is a response to distressful events. It is a protective response to negative events that threaten us, from vague apprehensions to gnawing anxieties, to overt dangers. The withdrawal response is a basic neuromuscular response to stress, just as Selye's general adaptation syndrome is a basic glandular response. Indeed, it is a specification of that response: that is, a protective response to negative stressors.

For example, when worries trigger this response, the eyes and forehead contract, wrinkling the skin. If we worry long enough, our skin becomes permanently wrinkled. When anxieties cause the neck muscles to flex, the face is projected forward in space, causing the muscles at the base of the neck (around the seventh cervical vertebra) to contract mightily, in order to hold up this forward-hanging burden. The more frequently this happens, the stronger and larger the muscles and fat tissue grow around the seventh cervical vertebra, thus creating what is called a dowager's hump.

It is the same with the shoulders, whose posterior surface is connected to the neck by the same trapezius muscles. When distressful events cause us to worry, they cause the reflex of lifting and rounding the shoulder blades forward. One cannot worry without contracting the shoulders. It is impossible to say, "Oi Veh!" without lifting the shoulders. That is why people with chronic worry often have chronically sore shoulders and necks. If serious worries afflict a human early enough in life, the stooped shoulders will occur early. It is a measure of childhood anxiety to what degree a child's shoulders are slumped and neck contracted. During the distressful teenage years, this posture is common.

Thus, it is not "age" that causes these bodily changes, it is distress. The more there is of it, and the longer it lasts, the more the Red Light reflex shows its long-term effects. It is not "age" that causes a stooped posture and shallow breathing; it is accumulated response to negative stress. Having a family and taking care of the kids and holding a job and paying the bills and solving the daily problems of life are all causes of looking old and stooped, unable to climb steps without getting breathless and hearing one's heart beat faster.

A stooped posture and shallow breathing go together. Both are caused by contraction of the abdominal muscle. The rectus abdominis is a long, powerful sheath of muscles that stretches from its lower attachments at the pubic bone and groin line all the way over the front of the chest and up to the nipple line. When it contracts, the upper part of the rib cage is pulled forward and down, and the pubic bone is pulled forward and up. The trunk is, thereby, pulled into the flexed curve of the fetal posture.

Contraction of the abdominal muscle not only depresses the rib cage, it depresses the entire contents of the abdominal cavity, creating pressure on the viscera. This means that when the diaphragm muscle between rib cage and abdomen contracts during inhalation, and begins to come downward toward the abdominal cavity, breathing is abruptly stopped. The pumplike downward movement of the diaphragm is necessary in order to create a vacuum in the thoracic cavity to draw in air. But if the impacted viscera inhibit this downward movement, no vacuum is created, and breathing is insufficient.

As we come to understand how the muscular contractions of the Red Light reflex cause bodily malfunctions, we acquire a different viewpoint on some of the common "maladies of old age." Not only does this abdominal contraction cause shallow breathing, it creates other problems as well. The pressure on the viscera affects all visceral functions. For example, when liquid pressure rises in the bladder, the urethra automatically contracts, giving us the urgent sense of needing to urinate. But when the abdominal muscle becomes contracted, it squeezes the bladder, raising its internal pressure, and giving the false sense of a full bladder. "Frequent urination" is a common complaint of older humans. It is usually the result of an habituated Red Light reflex. This same abdominal contraction affects digestion and elimination. Constipation and a chronically contracted stomach muscle often go together.

These are secondary effects of the withdrawal response. If one does not understand how they can cause basic malfunctions of the respiratory and digestive systems, the mistake is easily made that these are "medical problems"—indicating breakdown and degeneration of the internal organs. This is not necessarily the case. That is why these malfunctions may disappear when one learns to control the neuromuscular reflex creating them.

Aching legs and knees are typical of elderly persons. Careful observation reveals that these old persons have begun to walk with their knees slightly bent, so that the weight-bearing function of a straight knee is lost. If the thigh muscles are constantly engaged in weight support during waking, they will become chronically fatigued and sore. In addition, the areas under the kneecap and behind the knee joint, where the thigh tendons cross over the knee to attach to the lower leg, will become sore and sometimes inflamed. Arthroscopic surgery is not a likely solution. The solution, rather, lies in overcoming the Red Light reflex, in order to walk once again with the full support of a vertical leg.

There are many other malfunctions that result when the body is habitually contracted in the withdrawal response. These malfunctions are not typical medical diseases but something else: what Hans Selye termed "diseases of adaptation."[3] I agree with Selye. Such diseases would not occur if one had the ability to adapt to these stresses by the intelligent use of Somatic Exercises. The effect is that our muscles become free of the control of lower-brain reflexes and are returned to our voluntary control.

How the Withdrawal Response Becomes Habituated in Our Bodies

Habituation is the simplest form of learning. It occurs through the constant repetition of a response. When the same bodily response occurs over and over again, its pattern is gradually "learned" at an unconscious level. Habituation is a slow, relentless adaptive act, which ingrains itself into the functional patterns of the central nervous system.

When you see someone exhibit any or all of the postural distortions of the withdrawal response, you are looking at a posture that has been imprinted in the neuromuscular system by habituation. A person standing in the stooped posture of old age has acquired a "habit" of doing so. He or she has not "broken down," or degenerated, in bodily structure. Instead, the person has become maladapted in his or her neuromuscular habits. It is crucial to understand this, because, if the person's bodily structure has really finally broken down, there is little more we can do than to give him or her a cane or some form of brace. But if the person's stooped posture—and all the many ailments that can go with it— is a bad habit learned by dint of chance repetition, then it can be corrected. Voluntary muscular control, once possessed but momentarily quite forgotten, can be relearned.

A considerable amount of research has been done on the habituation of mammals to the withdrawal response. Because the central nervous system of all mammals, including human beings, is the same, this research is highly revealing. Results show just how the Red Light reflex stamps its imprint on human posture.

As a group, mammals are very different from other animals in the way their startle reflex functions. In lower animals, this reflex is all-or-nothing—it has no gradations. In humans and other mammals, however, the startle reflex is subject to levels of response from low all the way up to very high. This graded amplitude of response can be studied and calibrated exactly by measuring the degrees of muscle contractions that occur during startle. They depend on a number of factors, all of which are relevant to human beings. First of all, the degree of response depends on the other levels of the brain that overlie the brain stem and that can modulate its initial responses. A prime influence on the startle response is expectation. Because expectation is such an important factor, I devote an entire chapter to it later on. Expectation can either dampen or heighten the withdrawal response. For example, if laboratory animals are made to fear that something harmful might happen, their startle reaction is sharply higher when it happens than it usually is when they do not have this fear.

This phenomenon is universally recognized among humans. When children are told a scary story, and suspense builds, and someone comes up behind them and shouts "Boo!"—they may jump right out of their shoes. All theater and movie directors know that creating a sense of suspenseful expectation is how to startle the audience the most. After sufficient buildup, the stimulus is suddenly introduced, and the muscles of the audience contract. Everyone, because their withdrawal reflex has contracted the abdomen, pushing out the air, suddenly exclaims—"Oh!"

In contrast to this high-level startle response, humans can also undergo the same reaction at low levels—so low that the startle response can be picked up only by sensitive electrodes measuring the electrical activity of muscular contraction (electromyograms, EMG). In some fascinating research reported from Canada, it was found that EMG tension rose when a person was engaged in any challenging task involving fear of failure. When the task was completed, EMG tension fell back to normal levels.[4] In one experiment, EMG tension was recorded from the muscles of the forehead, which are very sensitive to the Red Light reflex. At the same time the subjects listened to a suspenseful detective story. As the story continued, the rise in muscular tension continued, making it clear to the researchers that feelings of suspense are directly tied to the feeling of muscular tension. When the story reached its climax, and the dangerous situation was dispelled, the tension that had been slowly building up dissolved abruptly, returning to its original level.

But there were some important exceptions. When the story was interrupted in the middle, the accumulated muscle tension remained, even hours later. The Canadian researchers discovered this phenomenon to be a general human trait: Tension built up during any human task involving fear of failure will not drop at its completion if there is no sense of completion. This concept can be quite subtle. If, at the end of a task, laboratory subjects are praised by the experimenter for their performance, their muscular tension drops. But if they are criticized, muscle tension remains. This is called "residual tension."[5]

According to research results from Canada, it is clear that the human neuromuscular system has the ability to adapt to a higher level of tension in these muscles, triggered by the withdrawal response. It is obvious that, if suspense and fear preexist, the startle response is triggered more easily. In one Canadian experiment, highly anxious patients were compared to normal persons in their startle response to a sudden loud noise. Even before the experiment, the EMG showed the muscles of the anxious patients to be more contracted than those of the calmer control group. When the startling sound was made, the difference between the two groups of subjects was not so much in their immediate reaction. It became clear in what happened afterward. The normal persons' muscles returned to their original state within half a second after the initial abrupt sound. The anxious persons' muscle tension not only remained high but continued to rise during the test.[6]

Unfortunately, to live in an "advanced society" is to live in a society that is rife with distress. Anxiety is the very currency of exchange in an industrial society. Everyone lives with suspenseful stories that are not completed. Everyone lives with fears that are overcome only to be replaced by new fears. Everyone has anxiety: anxiety over one's life, over one's family, over one's financial security, over one's place in the community, over the safety of one's house, over one's own safety in the streets, over the safety of the country, over the safety of the human race. And our jobs, and customers, and the banks, and the loan companies, and the Internal Revenue Service, and the newspapers, and the television news programs all feed this anxiety, so that it accumulates in our lives, layer upon layer, creating ever rising levels of habitual muscular tension in our jaws, eyes, brows, necks, shoulders, arms, chests, bellies, and legs.

This same abdominal contraction creates two other problems, which lie midway along a continuum from traditional psychological to physiological problems: namely, impotence and hemorrhoids. The chronic contraction, which pulls the chest wall downward toward the groin and pubic bone, does not stop at that point, but tautens all of the muscles lying at the bottom of the pelvis between the pubic bone and the coccyx, that is, the muscular sling called the perineum or "crotch." The Red Light reflex causes contraction in the perineal muscles through synergistic action. Contraction also occurs because of the increased pressure in the abdominal cavity, which causes the sphincter muscles of the urethra and the anus to reflexly contract. This chronic tightening around the blood vessels leading to the penis and clitoris prevents full blood flow and full innervation, thus preventing tumescence.

Impotence is common among persons chronically contracted in the abdominal-perineal area. And these same persons are, predictably, shallow breathers subject to anxiety feelings. The problem would seem to be a traditional psychological one, but it is not. It is more often a reflexive muscular problem in which control has been lost. Sensory-motor amnesia commonly underlies chronic impotence, and it is generally seen in older persons. But it is a habit, not a degeneration of "old age." And habits can be broken.

Because chronic abdominal-perineal contraction causes the anus to contract, its constant tension will not allow it to relax during defecation. This creates intolerable pressure in the anal sphincter, brutalizing the blood vessels and causing hemorrhoids. The medical advice not to "strain at the stool" is relevant but not particularly helpful, because it is impossible to defecate without applying greater internal abdominal pressure. The solution is clear: relief of the anal/perineal contraction, which, in effect, means relief from the Red Light reflex. One cannot relieve only one part of the reflex; one must relieve it all. Cutting, stretching, or chemically treating the anus will not solve the problem, because the problem is functional, not structural. The anal contraction is not the specific cause of hemorrhoids; rather, it is the specific effect of the Red Light reflex. Relief from the control of the Red Light reflex not only relieves the anal contraction but also enhances potency, deepens breathing, raises the chest wall, enhances heart function, and much more.

Effects of the Withdrawal Response on Breathing and Heart Functions

As noted earlier, the attention given to the effects of stress has been immense, but it has failed to focus on the role played by the neuromuscular system. The withdrawal response is a major muscular reaction to negative stress, and a fundamental feature of this reaction is the depression of breathing. Cardiovascular disease is a paramount health problem in contemporary society. So it is extraordinary that, in the research on stress and heart function, there is almost no attention paid to breathing.[7] Respiration is considered either unimportant or a minor variable in this research. This is profoundly disappointing, because, in a sense, the heart and lungs are the same organ.

Venous blood entering the right chambers of the heart flows directly through the filtering and oxygenating tissues of the lungs before entering the heart's left chambers. The right side of the heart is linked to the left side via its passages through the pulmonary vessels. The effects of respiration on heart function are obvious: One cannot even cough, sigh, gasp, or hold one's breath without causing an immediate change in coronary activities. But these effects have been ignored in scientific research. If we were to search for a reason for this, we might first look at the ignorance of the relation between stress and neuromuscular responses among scientific researchers. If Selye and other more recent researchers had known about it, more attention would have been paid to it later on, just as a matter of course.

People who do not fall under the sway of the Red Light reflex have a relatively uninhibited abdominal muscle. They are capable of diaphragmatic breathing, with the belly expanding to the front and sides during inhalation. This type of deep breathing has the following effects on cardiac function:

1. decreased heart rate

2. decreased cardiac output

3. reduced peripheral systolic blood pressure

4. regulation of the cardiovascular system by parasympathetic functions of the autonomic nervous system

5. regulation of the heartbeat by the ebb and flow of respiratory sinus arrhythmia[8]

Number 5 is the most universally recognized effect of respiration on cardiovascular function. Respiratory sinus arrhythmia refers to the way in which heart rate varies with the phase of respiration: The heart rate accelerates during the inspiratory phase, then decelerates during the expiratory phase. This alternation is a sign of how the parasympathetic branch of the autonomic nervous system dominates the stressed sympathetic branch, which governs the flight-or-fight response. The respiratory rate associated with this up-and-down rhythm is in the range of six breathing cycles a minute.

The five effects listed above characterize the unstressed cardiovascular functions that usually prevail during uninhibited diaphragmatic breathing. The respiratory sinus arrhythmia, with its rising and falling pressure, and its variable rate of flow, has the effect of massaging and buffing the vascular walls, which are flushed smooth by the pulsating pressure. The vascular canals tend, then, to remain supple.

The presence of respiratory sinus arrhythmia is a sign of coronary health; its absence is clinical evidence of a higher probability of coronary disease. It is known to be absent during sickness; moreover, we should not be surprised to discover that this healthy link between breathing and heart function usually diminishes with increasing age.

What takes its place? A steadier, nonvariable rate of heartbeat. And what else happens? The breathing rate is more rapid. And what psychophysiological state directly relates to this unhealthy change? Stress and the shallow breathing that occurs when the abdominal muscle tenses with the withdrawal response. As this response is repeated and its habituated effects accumulate during aging, breathing becomes shallower and more rapid. This is called hyperventilation.

A research study was carried out with 153 heart attack patients in the coronary care unit of a Minneapolis-St. Paul hospital.[9] These patients were examined to determine whether they were abdominal diaphragmatic breathers or thoracic breathers, whose tight abdominal muscles forced them into the labored chest-lifting characteristic of shallow breathers. The results of the survey were devastatingly clear: *Every single one of the 153 patients examined were thoracic breathers!*

Hyperventilation is a pattern of respiratory activity characterized by an increased ventilatory response. It is a condition that goes hand in hand with increased incidence of chest pains, heart palpitations, and the arterial narrowing of ischemia. It describes a Type A behavior characteristic seen in persons who are under increased risk of coronary heart disease.[10] It also seems to be directly linked to "essential" hypertension, that is, hypertension of no known cause. Of patients clinically diagnosed as hypertensive, from 80 to 95 percent show no known cause for their disease—such as kidney malfunction.[11]

However, given the evidence, we can surmise that there is indeed a cause, albeit a hidden one, of hyperventilation, one that has been neither particularly noticed nor investigated: the Red Light reflex, whose activation is endemic to industrial societies, and whose habituation causes the shallow thoracic breathing of hyperventilation. Hyperventilation has the following known effects on the heart:

1. increased heart rate

2. increased cardiac output

3. suppression of respiratory sinus arrhythmia and its replacement with a nonvarying heart rate

4. loss of parasympathetic control over cardiac functions and its replacement by sympathetic nervous functions

5. lowering of CO_2 arterial pressure and alteration of Ph, constricting both cerebral and skin blood vessels.

The two medical researchers who have explored these matters in the most thorough manner are Defares and Grossman. Their resumé of the scientific literature touching upon this crucial topic concludes with this statement:

Our analysis suggested some interesting possibilities for interventional strategies to reduce risk among Type A individuals. A breathing therapy oriented toward slowing down the respiratory pattern and increasing the depth of respiration might prove an effective means of treatment . . . . it is possible to alter the breathing pattern in a relatively stable manner. Such therapies might simultaneously reduce both psychological and coronary risk.[12]

The Somatic Exercises devised to counteract the effects of the Red Light reflex are just "such therapies." They enable us to remember what it feels like not to be anxious, and to breathe once again like healthy human beings are meant to breathe.

Chapter 9

The Green Light Reflex

The Back Muscles and the Action Response

People are always amazed to discover that they are doing things they are unaware of. This is because adults proudly hold on to the illusion that they are always conscious of what they are doing. For not to be conscious of what one is doing strikes one as a sign of incompetence, even irresponsibility. Nevertheless, these acts that we are oblivious of have major consequences in our lives. One of them, we now know, is the withdrawal response, when our abdomen, shoulders, and neck cringe in apprehension—the Red Light reflex. There is another response which also occurs constantly, but this time when we feel called upon, not to withdraw, but to act: the Green Light reflex.

The Green Light reflex could almost be thought of as necessary to industrial society, for to create an industrial economy, this reflex must be triggered constantly throughout the entire population. It is just as much a part of twentieth-century society as alarm clocks, calendars, coffee, quotas, sales commissions, and deadlines—each of which acts as a spur to this deeply embedded reflex.

In our society, 80 percent of the adult population suffer back pain. Apparently, the progress of technology is based on progressively deteriorating backs. This is ironic, because, in our contemporary technological society, the reward for escaping from back-breaking manual labor should be freedom from such physical pain. Compounding the irony, twentieth-century medicine has been spectacularly successful in extending our longevity to the limit our genes will allow. At the same time, however, it has been spectacularly unsuccessful in combating—even understanding—the epidemic we now see of chronic pain in the skull, neck, shoulders, back, and buttocks of the entire adult population. As René Caillet, a well-known specialist in medical rehabilitation, observes, "low back pain remains an enigma of modern society and a great dilemma for the medical profession."[1] It is the most common disorder for which people seek medical help. Moreover, it is the most common cause of worker absenteeism in industrial societies.[2] It is the general disorder for which the largest amount of money is spent on insurance and pharmaceutical and medical services—in the billions.

How can anything so painful, so epidemic, so socially detrimental, and so expensive be so little understood and so poorly coped with? How can medical researchers and practicing physicians, who study and treat back pain, be so unfortunate as to have the same pains in their backs? As a medical enigma, it is a cause of universal embarrassment.

The answer to this question touches upon something we have just mentioned: We constantly do things that have major consequences in our lives, yet we are quite oblivious to the fact that we are doing them. This is because, obviously, we cannot be aware of bodily events that are occurring unconsciously. What is more, we and our business leaders, social planners, and medical researchers—would be amazed to learn that we unconsciously cause our own pain. Not to be conscious of self-inflicted suffering may seem like a sign of incompetence and irresponsiblity, but the problem goes deeper than that.

We have not solved this problem, because we have not—until now—understood it. And we have not understood it, because the answer has been hidden from us, as it were, in the recesses of our consciousness; or, to be more precise, beneath the conscious control of the cerebral cortex, wherein voluntary movements originate. It lies hidden within the lower regions of the brain in a reflex that is so familiar, so unconscious, and so human that it is as invisible to us and yet ever present as the air we breathe. It is a reflex that is very specific in its function: It readies us for action. And, because we live in a world where programs of reliable and precisely scheduled actions are the necessary oil of the wheels of commerce, this reflex of ours is constantly being triggered until it has become habituated as part of our bodily functioning.

Without understanding the reflexive nature of these universal back disorders, we see this epidemic phenomenon as a scientific enigma. Caillet comments:

> An enigma remains in that there is no universality or standardization of low back pain disorders. The term "syndrome" must remain in today's terminology without clarification or universal understanding. Thus low back pain remains a symptom of vague etiology. Numerous terms prevail in the literature along with nonspecific mechanisms and, therefore, nonspecific treatment regimes. Terms such as lumbosacral strain, unstable back, lumbar discogenic disease, facet syndrome, pyriformis syndrome, iliolumbar ligamentous strain, quadratus lumbar pain, myofascitis, spinal stenosis, degenerative disc disease, latissimus dorsi syndrome, abnormal transforaminal ligaments, multifidus triangle syndrome, and a great many more enjoy current vogue.
>
> Each diagnosis is evaluated and treated with varying success. Treatment can include epidural steroid injection, manipulation, rhizotomy, electrocautery, chemical therapy, and facet joint injection, in addition to the time-honored standards of rest, posture training, traction, medication, and systematic exercise.[3]

In other words, medical confusion: shooting in all directions because one doesn't know what to aim at.

When health authorities display such confusion in face of a health problem affecting the majority of the population, they further compound the embarrassment when they attempt to explain away the problem. For a long time the medical world has supported the myth that back disorders are natural and inevitable.

This absurd yet widely spread unscientific notion is pithily summed up by Leon Root, M.D.: "What we can say without dispute is that the change in man from quadraped to biped, and the accompanying change in the structure of his back, is the main, if not exclusive, reason for the prevalence of low back pain among human beings."[4] Dr. Root pronounces such nonsense without fear of dispute. This is because, in the face of confusion, one must at least blame the problem on something—despite all that we know about mutation and natural selection and the enormous evolutionary advantage of the vertical human posture. And we would be wise not to lay the blame on God, or on evolution—neither is known for making mistakes in design. The human spinal column is a marvelous structure. It is designed so that its center of gravity is as high as possible, in order to allow for maximum mobility with the least expenditure of energy possible. Moreover, a vertical spinal column allows humans to walk, a feature that made possible the evolution of the unique human hand and brain.

It's easy to see that the myth about back disorders follows the same mistaken line of reasoning as does the myth about aging: Somehow, an "inevitable" structural breakdown is taking place. Both are false. The reason for the prevalence of back disorders is a breakdown not in the structure but in the function of the back. This is a crucial point. A broken structure cannot be made new again, but a disordered function can; moreover, it can even be improved.

The Landau Reaction and the Responsible Adult

In the first year of life an adventure is taking place. It is the discovery of the muscles of the back. And the most exciting moment of this adventure is the discovery of the Green Light reflex. When the Green Light reflex first springs into action, the tiny human is thrilled by the sensation of moving itself forward through space. This sensation, and the excitement of discovery that follows, continues throughout the entire span of human life.

At birth the infant is a helpless, cuddly mass of frontal flexing movements, which enable it to cling to the body of its mother. It cannot lift its head, arch its back, or support its trunk in sitting. Its back muscles are inoperative. During the first weeks, then, the human baby is one-sided: The muscles in the front of its body are highly active; the muscles in the back are highly inactive—they are, as it were, still asleep.

But not for long. Soon, by the third month, the baby does something astounding. Its little body begins to lift up its enormous head, as if this were the most important thing in the world. It is. The baby, when lying prone, is lifting its head so that its face will be vertical and its mouth horizontal. This allows the baby to learn two wonderful things: a sense of balance in the head and a sense of the horizon through the eyes. These are important, moreover, for reasons that are profoundly human. When the small head lifts and learns to level itself with the earth, the infant is teaching him or herself the first elements of the functions of standing and walking. These functions, genetically programmed, are thereafter pursued with great appetite.

Discovering how to lift and balance the head only whets the appetite for more adventure. The infant is now able to contract the muscles behind the neck but as yet is unable to contract those farther down the posterior of the body. Impatient wrigglings combine with the impatient unfolding of various genetic traits to bring the child to a triumphant achievement at about five months or so: He or she begins to arch the back. But that is not all. At the same time the baby learns to lift and straighten his or her arms and legs.

At this stage, five to six months, a new gravitational response has sprung into being: the Landau reaction (see Figure 16a). By holding the infant with one hand beneath its thorax and lifting it, not only does its head lift but—for the first time—its back arches and its legs extend. The muscles necessary for standing and walking come to life. This is the Landau reaction. It is a crucial stage of development for the young human. If it is absent at six months (see Figure 16b), it is a sign that something may be seriously wrong—for example, cerebral palsy. But if development is normal, from six months on, the human infant can perform a swimming movement on its stomach while lifting its head and moving its arms and legs. This is because it can now arch the powerful muscles of the lower back.

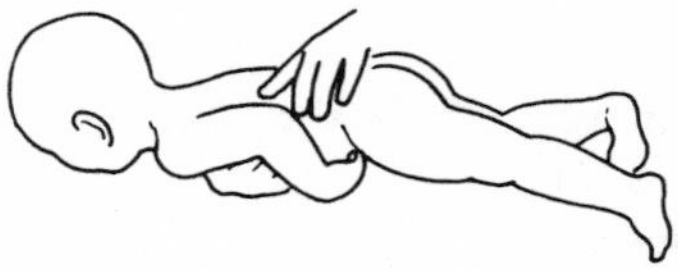

Figure 16a
The Landau Reaction

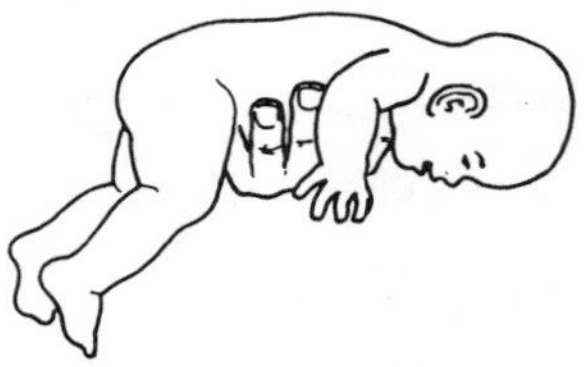

Figure 16b
Absence of the Landau Reaction

The Landau reaction means that the infant can now do something that is even more thrilling than "swimming." When it arches its back, straightening out its bent knees, it can push against the floor and thrust its head forward: in other words, it can now move itself through space! This is the full discovery of the Green Light reflex. Up until this point the infant more resembled a plant, rooted in one spot. But now the fledgling human being can not only move forward toward a goal but can even choose the goal, busily activating the back muscles and extending the legs in the newfound thrill of locomotion.

It is the contraction of the lower back muscles that inaugurates the Landau reaction. When the lumbar muscles connecting the back of the pelvis to the vertebrae contract, the infant has two simultaneous sensations: going up, and going forward. It is a delicious feeling. But this lumbar contraction is accompanied by the synergistic tensing of the muscles of the neck, shoulder, buttocks, and thighs. They, too, are part of the Landau reaction and are essential for the erect carriage of the body in standing and walking.

The Green Light reflex is the opposite of the Red Light reflex, as both a muscular activity and an adaptational function. The Red Light reflex contracts the anterior flexor muscles, curling the body forward; the Green Light reflex contracts the posterior extensor muscles, lifting and arching the back in the opposite direction. The adaptational function of the Red Light reflex is protective; it is a withdrawal from the world. The Green Light reflex is assertive; its function is action, and it too is adaptational. One makes us stop, the other makes us go. Thus, they are in balance, and are both necessary for our survival. They are equally necessary to our sense of well-being.

The activation of both these reflexes requires an expenditure of energy. Remembering Selye's statement, that stress is in response to good things as well as bad, we can say that both reflexes are stressful. If the Red Light reflex is negative distress, the Green Light reflex is positive, what Selye called eustress. The action response is, therefore, a positive form of energy expenditure.

From the sixth month onward, the Landau reaction grows stronger and stronger. Soon the child learns to turn over back to front and front to back. A baby girl can sit balanced at eight months and has already started to pull herself up to a standing position. By nine months, she can crawl on her hands and knees. Before long she is moving about on her hands and feet. By 10 months she can pivot and turn her body and walk holding on to furniture. Not long after that she is walking by herself. As soon as she does this, she wants to run! The world is now open to her, and the initial thrill of locomotion has expanded into an adventure of constant exploration and discovery.

From infancy through childhood and on through adolescence the young human is enormously active. The action response is triggered over and again as youngsters propel themselves into the world around them. The Green Light reflex, centered in the lower back, unconsciously precedes and prepares her for every positive action. Children are motivated to explore. Their activity is spontaneous and usually joyful. But as they grow, they begin to learn another reason for action: responsibility. They learn that there are some things they "have to do." They have to do their homework. They have to do their chores. They have to take baths, and they have to go to school. They have to perform more and more actions they are not spontaneously motivated to perform. They are learning what it means to become responsible adults.

Adults must make a living and be able to take care of themselves—whether they want to or not. The Green Light reflex is still being triggered, but the thrill is fast disappearing. The muscles of the back, now totally mastered, are being activated increasingly toward the responsibilities of life. The more responsible one is, the more often the back muscles are triggered.

We must recognize that the stressful aspects of aging begin early in life, usually in adolescence. The role of the adult differs among different cultures; some are more stressful than others. Within the industrial societies of the twentieth century, adulthood is highly stressful. Clocks, calendars, quotas, sales commissions, and multiple cups of coffee are all integral to the adult role. The general effect is that a great deal of stress is engendered. The specific effect is the habitual contraction of the muscles of the back.

In our society, most people begin to "get old" early in life. Our technology lets us live a long life, but it also condemns us to live out those years in discomfort and fatigue. An industrial society is fueled by the energy of the Green Light reflex, which is triggered incessantly. This relentless repetition guarantees that the muscular contractions of the reflex will be constant and habitual. The action response is so steady that, eventually, we cease to notice it. It becomes automatic, fading into oblivion. This is sensory-motor amnesia, and once it takes over we can no longer control the Green Light reflex. All we feel is fatigue, soreness, and pain—in the back of our heads, in our necks, our shoulders, upper back, lower back, and buttocks.

Chapter 10

The Sum of Neuromuscular Stress: The Senile Posture and the "Dark Vise"

Our examination of the muscular reflex patterns incurred by stress has produced a fundamental insight: There are two major reflexes triggered by stress. Together, they account for a major portion of the physiological malfunctions that typically occur as humans age.

The Red Light reflex and the Green Light reflex (see Figures 17 and 18) are, as basic adaptive reflexes, deeply inscribed in our central nervous system. A correct appreciation of the roles of these two major reflex patterns gives a more complete understanding of the stress response initially developed by Hans Selye. In so doing, it allows us to understand why the quality of what happens to us during the years of our life is infinitely more crucial to our health and happiness than the quantity of how many years we have lived our lives.

These two adaptive reflexes are essential to our survival as a species and as individuals. They serve, respectively, to protect us from danger in the world, and to move us toward the opportunities of the world. They are as necessary to our lives as the air we breathe and the food we eat.

The typical problems that occur during human aging are due to the combined effect of the withdrawal response and the action response. In comparing these two muscular responses (see Figures 17 and 18), you will see that they oppose each other, pulling in opposite directions to serve the opposite functions of protection and mobility. They are total somatic responses; that is, not only do they involve the entire musculature from head to toe, but also engage the entire central nervous system in a specific orientation of either negative withdrawal or positive action. If we view it objectively, we see only the movement of musculature; but more is happening subjectively: A specific feeling and set of sensations accompany this muscular movement.

When either of these opposing reflexes occurs, it affects the body's entire musculature. Almost every muscle has an opposite muscle that counterbalances it. Each agonist has an antagonist, so that, for example, when we contract our biceps to flex our arm, the triceps extensor muscle, its antagonist, automatically relaxes. Thus, in the Red Light reflex, the front half of the body's musculature contracts, while its antagonist, the back half, relaxes and lengthens. This means that all of the muscles in the whole body—all agonists and antagonists—are simultaneously involved.

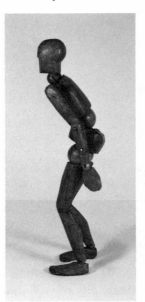

Figure 17   The Red Light Reflex
From head to toe, the Red Light reflex involves the following movements: closing eyes, tensing jaw and face, pulling forward of neck, lifting of shoulders, flexing elbows, clenching fists, flattening chest, tightening abdominal muscle, contracting diaphragm and holding breath, contracting perineum (including sphincters of anus and urethra), contracting gluteus minimus muscles to rotate thighs inward (feet are pigeon-toed), adduction of thighs, contraction of hamstrings to bend knees, flexing and supination of feet (each foot lifts and inverts, tilting up arch). The sensory feedback of all these movements constitutes the subjective feeling of the Red Light reflex: fear.

Figure 18   The Green Light Reflex
From head to toe, the Green Light reflex involves the following movements: opening eyes, jaw and face, pulling backward of neck, pulling downward of shoulders, extending elbows, opening hands, lifting chest, lengthening abdominal muscle, relaxing diaphragm and freeing breathing, relaxing anal and urethral sphincters in the perineum, contracting gluteus maximus muscles to extend thighs, contraction of gluteus medius muscles to rotate thighs outward (feet are ducklike), abduction of thighs, contraction of thigh extensors to straighten knee to hyper-extension, extension and pronation of feet. The sensory feedback of all these movements constitutes the subjective feeling of the Green Light reflex: effort.

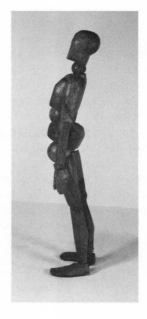

But this ideal seesaw balance between agonistic contraction and antagonistic relaxation is not what usually develops as we age. As the young human matures, various threatening and inviting situations will trigger the Red Light and Green Light reflexes many times. As these repetitions accumulate, each reflex pattern gradually becomes habitual. At first, it's only to a small degree, but, if frequency and intensity increase, the contractions become well established. Gradually, the Red Light and Green Light reflexes interfere with one another. When one is partially contracted, the other cannot contract fully.

This is the sum of neuromuscular stress, a state of muscular immobility caused by the gradual buildup of chronically opposing contractions.

The senile posture in Figure 19c is the summation of the two opposing reflexes (Figures 19a and 19b). It is a very familiar posture, seen in millions of aged bodies, and it clearly shows how the two reciprocal reflexes habituate into a tense compromise between the two patterns. The powerful contraction of the spinal muscles in the Green Light reflex continues its pulling of the lower back and neck into a curve. But the equally powerful pull of the abdominal and shoulder contractions in the Red Light reflex tilts the entire trunk forward, rounding the back and shoulders and projecting the head forward.

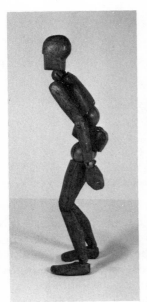

Figure 19a
Red Light Reflex

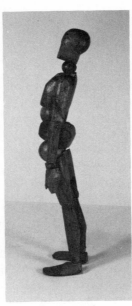

Figure 19b
Green Light Reflex

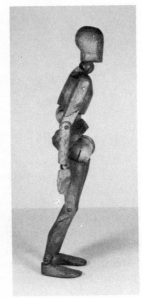

Figure 19c
Senile Posture

All three postures are shown in their extreme form, so we can clearly recognize them. In reality, however, because the human body is so variable, these postures occur in numerous combinations. Sometimes the Red Light reflex is much more dominant, creating a far more stooped posture of senility. Or the Green Light reflex may dominate, exaggerating the curves of the lower back, rib cage, and neck. Whatever the combination, the competition between the two reflexes gradually distorts the body in the direction of the senile posture. Although this occurs as the human being typically ages, it is the sum of habitual responses to neuromuscular stress that is the cause of the pathologies discussed in the following paragraphs.

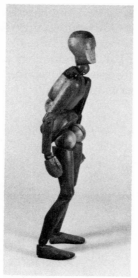

Figure 20a
Senile Posture
with Dominance of the
Red Light Reflex

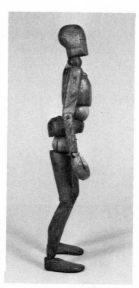

Figure 20b
Senile Posture
with Dominance of the
Green Light Reflex

1. Stiff and limited movements.   As the Red Light and Green Light reflexes close in on one another, the human skeleton becomes imprisoned within its own musculature. As noted earlier, it is the muscles around the body's center of gravity that are the central agents of both reflexes. As they simultaneously pull the pelvis and hips up toward the trunk, yet pull the trunk and shoulder girdle down toward the pelvis, all movements become limited. The free rotational movement between the pelvis and the trunk is restricted. This automatically restricts walking. The pelvis doesn't swing, and the arms lose their counter-swing to pelvic rotation. Rather than the right arm coming forward with the left leg (Figure 21a), it begins to come forward with the right leg. The trunk has become rigid, like a single block (Figure 21b).

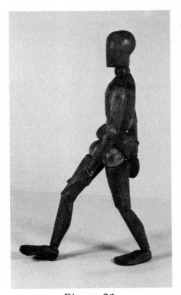 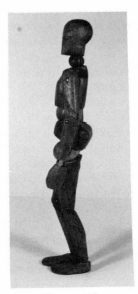

Figure 21a	*Figure 21b*
Walking with Counterswing	Walking with Rigid Trunk

Both the arms above the trunk and the legs below the pelvis are similarly restricted, as is the head. As the senile posture develops, it becomes impossible to turn the head all the way around, for example, to look behind you when you try to park the car. The shoulder girdle is pulled downward, preventing the arms from reaching and rotating. Women have trouble putting on their brassieres, and golfers have trouble following through with a full swing. It becomes difficult to turn the knees in and out in free rotation. Dancing is too much of an effort. It's hard to maintain balance, and a fear of falling develops, which, in turn, causes people to become more cautious and stiff in their movement.

2. Chronic pain. The chronically stiff contraction of the body's musculature causes a chronic ache in these same muscles. They become sore, sometimes genuinely painful. Because the early Landau reaction is being constantly trig-gered in the Green Light reflex, the discomfort in the muscles in the lower back and pelvic region will range from a dim ache to a lively pain, depending upon the degree of stressful activity. Moreover, the restrictions of the shoulder and hip joints will cause varying degrees of discomfort, depending upon the kind of habitual activities engaged in. Typists, for example, will have sore shoulders and necks; postal workers will have sore buttocks and hips. When the senile posture is well advanced, and the central body has become quite rigid, pain will begin in the extremities. It is this pain—for example, in the elbows and hands, or in the knees and feet—that physicians frequently mistake for arthritis, pinched nerves, carpal tunnel syndrome, and so on.

3. Chronic fatigue.   Inasmuch as the overlapping contractions of two reflexes simultaneously activate all of the body's muscle system, the result is an enormous expenditure of energy. One of the most common complaints of elderly humans is that they are always tired. "Please, can you do something to give me more energy?" is a plea I have heard hundreds of times. But these people do not lack energy. That is not their problem. Their problem is that, involuntarily and unconsciously, they are expending large amounts of energy constantly. These chronic contractions continue unabated when they are lying down, even during sleep. When they get up in the morning, they are dismayed to discover that not only do their muscles ache but they are tired as well. Some become so fatigued that they need to rest within an hour or two after rising.

Sometimes the subjective feeling is not of fatigue but of weakness. Frequently I read medical reports that state that the muscles of an elderly patient have become "weak." This is usually incorrect. If doctors would trouble to feel the affected muscles, they would discover that they are rigidly held in a tonic, involuntary contraction. They are, in fact, not weak, but strong, from their constant contraction. Often they become quite large and powerful from their chronic pulling.

4. Chronic shallow breathing.   The senile posture, by combining the contractions of the withdrawal and action responses, pulls down the entire rib cage, both front and back, immobilizing the chest. We have seen how this provokes the shallow, rapid breath of hyperventilation and its unfortunate effects on cardiovascular functions. When oxygen intake becomes extremely low, the result is often depression, listlessness, and loss of mental acuity.

5. A negative self-image.   When individuals reach a stage in life when (1) they can no longer do what they once did, (2) they are always in pain, (3) they are tired and without energy, and (4) their oxygen supply is restricted, these individuals usually develop a negative self-image. This may happen if, despite all their efforts, they cannot reverse the loss of their youthful functions, and if they constantly are told, "That's the inevitable effect of aging." This state of affairs has its own disastrous consequences, because, according to the somatic law, what you expect is usually what you get. This will be discussed in Chapter 12.

6. Chronic high blood pressure and the "Dark Vise."   Perhaps the major cause of death from diseases late in life is arteriosclerosis, also called "hardening of the arteries." This condition is at the root of both coronary and cardiovascular diseases, the latter of which include strokes and ruptured aneurysms. The scientific view of gerontological researchers is that high blood pressure, combined with hardening of the arteries which restricts blood flow, is what causes these events, and that this condition is the result of a genetically programmed biological process.[1] In other words, the medical view is that hypertensive arteriosclerosis is "the inevitable effect of aging."

But quite possibly it is not, and I say this for two reasons, one of which I have already mentioned in our discussion of the Red Light reflex: When the Red Light reflex restricts breathing and therefore triggers hyperventilation, it also suppresses the normal variable heart rhythm and pressure of sinus arrhythmia. This means that two things occur: (1) Dominance of the sympathetic nervous system over cardiovascular functions causes the smooth muscle walls of the vascular canals to contract; and (2) the up-and-down variation of blood pressure no longer occurs, so that the vascular walls are not kept supple and therefore adaptable to blood pressure changes.

The other reason for modifying the current viewpoint about the inevitability of hypertensive arteriosclerosis has to do with the known effects of static muscle contraction—also known as isometric contraction. There are two ways in which muscles can work: statically or dynamically. When you squeeze the juice from an orange, the fingers close down around the orange; this movement of the fingers is a dynamic contraction. When you squeeze a baseball, the fingers do not move, even though the muscles are contracting; this is static contraction.

Static contraction of muscles is what happens in isometric exercise, once made popular through the muscular development program of Charles Atlas. It is the contraction of one muscle group against another, as when one presses the palms of the hands tightly together causing the chest muscles to contract—the hands do not move, but the muscles do.

But there is a problem with this form of exercise: It causes a sharp rise in blood pressure.

> For the normal heart isometric exercise poses a unique stress. Unlike dynamic exercise, where cardiac output increases dramatically with typically no change in mean blood pressure, *during isometric exercise* cardiac output increases only slightly but *mean blood pressure increases* dramatically. *This results in a sharp increase in the afterload on the heart. . . .* The increased afterload associated with isometric exercise has been *shown to precipitate many of the symptoms of congestive heart failure* in many individuals with a diseased myocardium.[2]

It is well known that blood pressure can increase up to 50 percent after isometric contraction.[3] The dangers posed by static muscle contraction are not limited to the heart; there is as well the risk of stroke and ruptured aneurysm. J. S.

Petrofsky, who has devoted an entire volume to a review of the research in this area, concludes his views about the effect of isometric exercise by warning that "it is apparent that this form of exercise would be dangerous for the elderly hypertensive patient."[4]

If we reflect upon the collision of the Red Light and Green Light reflexes in the senile posture and their statically opposing contractions, we suddenly realize the potential fatality of the senile posture. The body's two major muscle groups are opposing one another involuntarily in a static, isometric contraction—a Dark Vise that causes chronically high blood pressure. As mentioned above, hypertensive arteriosclerosis is at the root of cardiovascular disease, a major cause of death in later life. Moreover, it is common for elderly humans to have high blood pressure. By putting these two facts together, we come up with a cause of hypertensive arteriosclerosis: the senile posture that occurs due to the unimpeded habituation of the Red Light and Green Light reflexes. If these reflexes occur often enough and strongly enough, they can become habituated, fading gradually from voluntary consciousness into sensory-motor amnesia—and the Dark Vise takes over.

These six pathologies are the sum of neuromuscular stress in the lives of all human beings. They are the result of reflexes that are utterly normal and can do us no harm unless we cease to notice their occurrence and allow them to become so familiar that they become unconscious and habitual. These six pathologies are, then, avoidable: they are not "inevitable," which is to say that the major effects of aging are both avoidable and/or remediable.

I think it is horrifying to consider old age as a disease. It is equally horrifying to presume that a long life is a disease process with inevitable consequences. These six pathologies associated with typical aging do not comprise a disease; they are a syndrome, best described as the "aging syndrome." This means that they are the associated signs and symptoms of an unhealthy process that must be attended to and reversed.

Human beings are not in the least helpless. We can avoid, or dispel, the effects of the two neuromuscular responses to stress. We cannot avoid the responses themselves, because they are built into our genes. But we can be aware of them. We cannot always avoid the situations that cause them to occur, but we can control our responses to them. In animals, the withdrawal response and the action response are conditioned reflexes; recall Pavlov's dog, that salivated when it heard the bell ring. They may also become conditioned in us, but only if we think of ourselves as no different from Pavlov's dog.

Pavlov and many other physiologists have "scientifically" viewed the human being as just another animal. The somatic point of view, however, is profoundly different. According to somatics, the human is not just another animal—a more complex version of a laboratory rat. A human being is a self-aware being, capable of learning even greater self-awareness and greater self-control. Once we recognize the power of self-awareness, we know we can save ourselves from the inescapable forces of stress. Not to recognize the fact and utility of human consciousness would be to condemn ourselves, in effect, to live and die like dogs.

I do not think it is of the least importance whether science in general or medicine in particular recognizes the factual power of human self-awareness. By its own definition of human beings as animals, science precludes recognition of it. I do think, however, that it is of the highest importance that individuals—you and I—recognize it and put it to use. Not only would we avoid the avoidable pathologies that can occur during a long life, we would confirm to ourselves the power of human self-responsibility and autonomy—a power that has much deeper significance.

Interlude: **The Archer's Bow and The Danger of a "Tight Gut"**

When a person can't get rid of hiccups, everyone has a different remedy: "Put a paper bag over your head and rebreathe the exhaled air." "Drink water upside down." "Hold your breath till you can't hold it any longer." Sometimes these methods work. Usually they don't.

It is exactly the same when you have back pains. Friends as well as health professionals have an assortment of methods to suggest. Sometimes they work. Usually they don't. "Your back is too weak; you have to strengthen it." "Your back is too tight; you have to stretch it; touch your toes." "Your disks are herniated; you need an operation." "Your disks are bulging; you need a back brace." "All you have to do is sit with a swayback." "All you have to do is sit with a flat back." "It's very simple; when the back is too tight, it means the stomach muscles have become weak and flabby; tighten up your gut; that will solve the problem." Almost everyone has back problems, but they cannot help themselves, because they don't understand what has gone wrong. That's why their "solutions" are unsuccessful. The situation would seem comic if there were not so much pain and anguish involved.

In 99 percent of the cases of lower back pain, the pain is located in the muscles connecting the spine and rib cage to the back of the pelvis. The pain will be in the lower back or the pelvis or both, sometimes on both sides and sometimes on one side only. The muscles are painful for a single reason: excessive contraction, caused by the Green Light reflex.

Even a person with a comfortably functioning back can have lower back pain if he or she spends 10 hours in the field digging potatoes or picking cotton. The extensor muscles will become exhausted from repeatedly lifting up the trunk. But a person can also sit in a chair all day working at a desk or typewriter stand and have the same pain if the extensor muscles are constantly contracted by an habituated Green Light reflex. The spinal muscles in the lower back will be very firm and will pull the lower back into an arch. The painful swayback that afflicts most adults in our society is like an archer's bow. The muscles at the back of the spine are like the thong of the bow. When the thong is not taut, there is only a slight bend (Figure 22a), but when the thong is tightened, the bow is arched (Figure 22b).

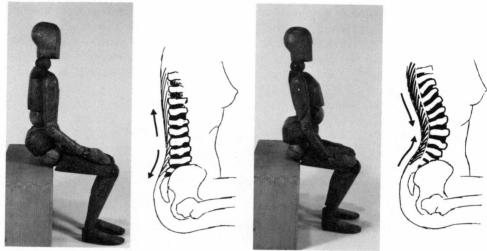

Figure 22a
Relaxed Spine

Figure 22b
Archer's Bow Spine

When the extensor muscles of the back are chronically contracted, the posture of the lower spine is bowed forward into an arch, which projects the belly forward and reduces the height of the trunk. The spinal column shortens, because a curved line is shorter than a straight line. This arch squeezes the back portions of the vertebrae down against the posterior sections of the spongy disks, which, being elastic like a golf ball, are compressed down pinching the posterior section, causing it to bulge out into the spinal canal (Figure 22b). Since X rays do not show muscle tissue (the tight "thong") but only the vertebrae and thick disks (the "bow"), radiologists frequently mistake the outward bulge of the disk for a collapse (hernia or rupture). Thus, they incorrectly assume that the vertebral structure has "broken down."

This mistaken image of a broken-down back haunts everyone's thinking about this universal problem. "Back-breaking labor" expresses this confusion as does the equally popular complaint, "My back went out." Except with fractures and severe accidents, human backs rarely "break" or "go out." They do, however, become painfully bent into the archer's bow, with the pain usually being in the constantly fatigued muscles of the back, not in the disks or in the nerves, as is commonly believed. If the sensory nerves in the lower back under the fourth and fifth lumbar vertebrae are pinched by excessive contraction, the pain will be felt, not in the back, but in the pelvis and leg on the side of the pinch. These are sciatic pains, which are an aggravated example of the same provisional compression of the disks into an archer's bow.

Because the archer's bow curves the lower back inward, it automatically curves the belly outward. "No matter how much I diet, I can't get rid of this protruding stomach!" is a remark of many middle-aged clients. Even though this protrusion is the unavoidable consequence of chronically contracted back muscles, there is a befuddled conviction among some health professionals that the back and belly sway forward because the abdominal muscles have become weak. Having a "tight gut" is an obsession with many males, and they will engage in long sessions of sit-ups and leg-lifts to remedy this situation. But nothing changes, because the abdominal muscles were never weak. Instead, the lower back muscles are excessively contracted—they are "too strong."

The typical curve in the middle of the body, then is, due neither to a "weak back" nor to a "weak belly"—nor is it due to a structural breakdown that must be repaired, braced, or trussed up. It is due to a chronic involuntary contraction of the back muscles caused by a constantly triggered Green Light reflex. The problem is in the brain where the reflex is habituated. When this reflex is mastered, the curved back, the protruding belly, the compressed disks all disappear—and the pain ceases. But sensory-motor amnesia causes us to forget what it feels like to have a relaxed, undistorted back. After years of suffering the effects of a curved and shortened spine, one's sense of "straight" is distorted.

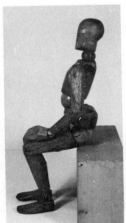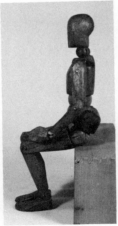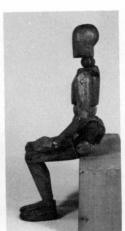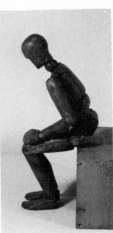

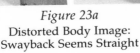
Figure 23a
Distorted Body Image:
Swayback Seems Straight

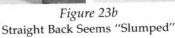
Figure 23b
Straight Back Seems "Slumped"

During the last 10 years I have never known a client with a painfully swayed back who, when he or she learned to release these muscles, failed to say, "But this doesn't feel straight. If feels slumped forward! If I am to sit up straight, I have to hold my back like this . . ." Whereupon they will contract and arch their lower back into the old curve, protruding the belly forward and pulling the head behind the center of gravity. In Figures 23a and 23b you see this crucial—and also fascinating—phenomenon of a distorted body image. In Figure 23a you see the distorted body image (dotted line) of a typically chronic Green Light reflex: the backward curve of the trunk seems "straight," so that when one first learns to relax back to a straight spine, it seems "slumped" (see Figure 23b). It takes a few weeks to become accustomed to having a tall undistorted back. It is crucial to keep this in mind as you begin to relax your back muscles in the first two Somatic Exercises.

Chapter 11

Trauma: The Role of Injury

When the Body Tilts

One question I always ask my clients is whether they have had any bone fractures, serious accidents, surgery, or any other cause for hospitalization. Another thing I always do is look at the person head-on to see if he or she is tilting to the side. Sometimes I ask the person to walk, to see if there is any hint of a limp. Both the questions and the observations are directed at achieving the same goal: to determine if there have been any traumatic injuries.

The gradual effects of the habituated Red Light and Green Light reflexes on the body are most easily seen from the side: that is, the swayed back and protruding belly of the archer's bow posture or the stooped upper trunk of the *viejito*. But the sudden effects of trauma are best seen head-on from the front or from the back: that is, the sideways tilting of the trunk. Long-term stress affects the body on both sides equally, but it does not cause tilting. But trauma will affect the body only on the side where the injury occurred, causing the muscles to cringe and curve the body to one side.

The trauma reflex is a reaction of the sensory-motor system meant to guard against pain. It is a common protective reflex, as transparently familiar as the breath-holding crouch of the Red Light reflex or the arching back of the Green Light reflex. When we are stung by a bee or pricked by a hypodermic needle, we flinch—that is the trauma reflex. If someone holds a burning cigarette or a sparkler too near to us, we move the threatened body part away from the danger and cringe—that is the trauma reflex. If our body is injured, the muscular cringing is meant to hold a tight protective pattern around the point of injury—that too is the trauma reflex.

These kinds of trauma reflexes can occur in any part of the body—top or bottom, front or back, left or right side. They can occur in the front of the body, adding to the contracted crouch of the Red Light reflex, as happens sometimes after heart surgery. They can occur in the back of the body, adding to the tight swayback of the Green Light reflex, as sometimes occurs after spinal surgery. But unless the injury is in the center of the body, the cringing contraction of the trauma reflex will be most obviously seen on one side of the body, usually affecting the smoothness of walking and the sense of balance.

When there is scoliosis, it means that trauma has occurred. Orthopedic physicians frequently ignore trauma as a factor in a child's scoliosis, sometimes propounding the outlandish theory that the causes are genetic, that one side of the body grows faster than the other! In the tiniest fraction of cases this might, indeed, occur, but usually such genetic deformities occur along with other signs of deformity—something rarely the case with scoliosis.

Scoliosis can be a simple curve like a long C, or it can be a double curve like an S (Figures 24a and 24b). In the latter case, the lower spine is curved in one direction and the thoracic spine is curved in the opposite direction. The genesis of this is usually always the following: An injury occurs on one side of the body, causing the muscles of the pelvis and lumbar spine to contract tighter on one side, but the righting reflex of our balancing system automatically pulls the head and upper trunk in the opposite direction to counterbalance the lower tilt. In Figures 24a and 24b you see the effect of reflexive muscle contraction over which the person has lost control; that is, SMA has occurred. Whether the curve is simple or S-shaped, the cause is usually the same: trauma to one side of the body, causing reflex muscular contraction.

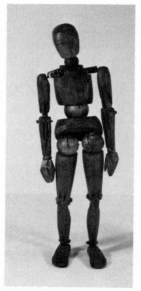

Figure 24a
Simple Scoliosis with C Curve

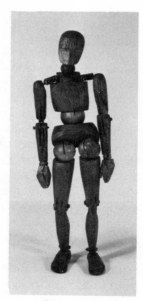

Figure 24b
Scoliosis with S Curve

The trauma reflex can be triggered by any severe damage to the body. In the case histories of Part 1, Barney, who leaned heavily to the right, had broken his left thigh in an automobile accident three years earlier; Louise's "frozen" right shoulder and right tilt occurred after she had fallen, breaking her upper arm; Harley had fallen out of a truck, injuring his left knee. Thereafter he limped, leaning to the left.

The trauma reflex can be triggered by surgery: A spastic cringing reaction will occur in the muscles surrounding the site of surgery. Women who have mastectomies may have chronic stiffness and soreness in the shoulder and upper rib cage. Men who have heart surgery may have a tight soreness in the chest. People who have kidney surgery and a catheter insertion will sometimes have uncontrollable muscular spasms in the lower belly and upper thigh where the catheter had been. Examples of this kind are endless.

Equally frequent are trauma reflexes on one side of the body after a severe fall on the hip, or following a sprained ankle or a broken leg. The inability to put weight on the injured leg causes an automatic shift of weight to the other leg. This is not a voluntary action; it is a reflex to avoid the pain. One cannot help but "favor" the injured leg. Tailors as well as chiropractors will frequently tell their clients that one of their legs is shorter than the other. Out of hundreds of persons who have been told that, I have never seen one whose leg was actually shorter; in every case, the muscles of the center of the body were chronically contracted, pulling up the hip on the side—like Harley's "retracted landing gear." There are as many varieties of the trauma reflex as there are ways for humans to injure themselves, ranging from the bruskly to the subtly violent and from a whiplash twist of the neck to a paralytic disease.

Inequality between the two sides is so common that we see it constantly but do not notice it. In fact, curved spines are so "normal" that few health practitioners realize that persons tilted to one side by accident will, if their lower back becomes increasingly arched by the Green Light reflex, risk pinching one or both of their sciatic nerves.

Sciatica is caused by disk pressure on the sciatic nerves located just between the fourth and fifth lumbar vertebrae and the fifth lumbar vertebra and the first sacral vertebra, respectively. They are sensory nerves, extending through the pelvis, down the thigh and calf, ending in the foot. The former goes down the side of the leg, ending in the big toe; the latter goes down the back of the leg to the heel, ending in the little toe. Whichever nerve is pinched, the pain will be felt along that route. If the pinch is moderate, the pain is felt only in the pelvis and hip. If the pressure is severe, the pain is like a hot wire going all the way to the foot. It is a nerve pain with a different sensation than muscular pain, and it can be agonizingly debilitating when it is severe.

Except in obvious cases of severe accidents and compression fractures, sciatica is a relatively common adaptive disease. Like all diseases of adaptation, it is directly related to the amount of stress and trauma that has occurred in that person's life. The longer we live, the more chance we have to experience stress and trauma; therefore, sciatica is often associated with the diseases of aging. But it can occur at any age. And as a disease of adaptation, sciatica can be either avoided or remedied. Teaching people how to avoid or get rid of the sciatic condition has been one of the more interesting aspects of my work as a somatic educator. I am frequently consulted by persons with severe sciatica who are desperate to avoid surgery.

A baker in his early forties hobbled into my office with excruciating sciatic pains down his left leg to the big toe. He was terrified of the pain, but more terrified of the back surgery that was considered "necessary." After a few sessions, he regained sensation and motor control of the lumbar and left trunk muscles. The pain then disappeared, first in the leg, then in the back. The intervertebral disk that was presumed to be "ruptured" had, as it turned out, merely been bulging from the viselike pressure of involuntary contraction in the lower back muscles. With the contractions now under his voluntary control, the vertebrae returned to their normal position. To perpetually celebrate the fact that his back is perfectly sound, he now makes a great show of lifting 100-pound sacks of flour to pour into his mixing machine. He has been doing this for three years.

In another instance, I worked with a cowboy who was out of rodeo competition because of chronic sciatic pain. Ten days after our last of three sessions of retraining, he was at San Francisco's Cow Palace bronco-busting and steer riding at the Grand National competition.

It is this near-miraculous capacity of the human consciousness and the central nervous system to learn and adapt that is the theme of this book. We are capable of far more than we believe ourselves to be. As we learn more and more about the ways in which brain functions control, maintain, repair, and protect our bodies, we come more and more to respect this marvelous capacity we have. We are far less dependent and helpless than we believe ourselves to be; which is to say, we are far more responsible and self-governing than we know.

Interlude: **Staying Sexy and Smart**

A common myth of aging is that, after the first flush of youth, we steadily begin to lose both our sexual and our mental competence. But this is not what really happens.

There is, however, an element of truth to the myth of declining sexual competence, and it has to do with males and with the high frequency of orgasms possible when they are four years into adolescence. This initial explosion of sexuality drops, by the end of the teenage period, to a relatively steady state, which continues at such a stable level that, at 50-plus years, 98 percent of men are still sexually active.

Our knowledge about early sexuality comes from Alfred C. Kinsey's groundbreaking reports of some three decades ago. But Kinsey's survey only included persons up to 65 years old, and the number sampled at the 50-plus level was minimal. This missing information was richly supplied in 1984 with the publication of the Consumers Union report, *Love, Sex, and Aging*,[1] which covered the age span of the 50s through the 80s. This report on 4,246 respondents covered the largest geriatric sample ever assembled for a sexuality study.

What this report tells us is that the decline in sexual competence in later years is minimal: The frequency may not be that of the late teenager, but, if we peruse the report's personal remarks, the pleasure is apparently greater. It seems that older persons need fewer repetitions to do it right.

The sexual responsiveness of women reaches its fullness considerably later than that of males, that is, during their late twenties and early thirties. The average frequency of female sexual activity remains fairly constant up until their sixties. Of all women in their fifties sampled in the Consumers Union report, 93 percent were sexually active. When we match this with the 98 percent of sexually active 50-year-old males sampled, we have a picture of human beings at the half-century mark whose sexuality does not subscribe to the myth of aging.

Given the known muscular discomforts and limitations of the average citizen after a lifetime of stress and accidental traumas, these are astonishing figures. It is just as astonishing that 91 percent of men in their sixties were sexually active, as well 81 percent of women. (Keep in mind that this reduced percentage includes many widows.) Surely by the time the average man or woman manages to reach their seventies they must be sexually exhausted. Not at all: 79 percent of all men and 65 percent of all women surveyed were still sexually active.[2]

So there is a decline in sexuality as humans age, but it is only a small decline. And, if humans could learn how to ward off the cumulative effects of stress and trauma in their nervous systems, there might be literally no decline at all.

Most impressive was the Consumers Union report on people in their eighties. Roughly half of these men and women were still sexually active, and the majority still rated the sexual experience as "very enjoyable." When asked what she had to say to younger people regarding love and sexual relationships, an 83-year-old San Diego woman replied, "That sex relations may continue indefinitely." A 68-year-old-widower wraps it up with this remark: "To sum up succinctly, I indulge less and enjoy it more. . . ."[3]

The myth about aging and sexuality has its parallel in false assumptions about aging and mental competence. When the Binet intelligence tests were first used in the United States, it was believed that intellectual development, running parallel with sexual development, reached a peak at age 16. During the 1920s, some researchers thought the peak might be even earlier, at perhaps 13 years. After these peaks, no further intellectual development was presumed to take place. (This is when the popular myth probably got its start.) But the Wechsler tests of the 1930s quickly revealed that the findings of the Binet tests were not true. According to the later tests, many adults seemed to get smarter as they got older. And the Wechsler scales turned up an interesting complication: Different types of intellectual function had different times and rates of peaking and declining. This was further complicated by the discovery that some adults did not show any decline at all.

We are all familiar with the way some elderly people say, "I'm not as sharp as I used to be," or "I don't have the head for it anymore," just as we know some elders have the memory dysfunction of Alzheimer's disease. Given the rapid change of each generation during the twentieth century, we are also familiar with the way the younger generation seems to be getting smarter than the older one. But is this due to a difference in age or to something quite separate: a difference in culture and education?

There was no way of definitely answering this question until a difficult scientific task could be attempted: to launch a "longitudinal study," which measured the intellectual abilities of a single group of people throughout their later adulthood. Keeping track of a large group of persons and retesting them over a 20- to 30-year period is a formidable task, and only a few such studies have been completed. Eight were published in a unique research report—*Longitudinal Studies of Adult Psychological Development.*[4] Its editor was K. Warner Schaie, whose own 21-year Seattle longitudinal study is the backbone of this book.

Schaie's study began with 1,656 subjects aged 25 through 67, tested in the years 1956, 1963, 1970, and 1977. This group was tested and retested for the growth or decline of various intellectual abilities. It became obvious that intellectual development did not peak at 16 years. Different intellectual abilities took different lengths of time to mature. For example, the ability to think with numbers does not reach its peak until age 32; reasoning ability peaks at 39; speech and word fluency do not hit their peaks until age 46; and comprehension of verbal meaning does not reach its stride until 53 years.[5] Apparently aging is not a period of decline but one of improvement and development. This was a stunning discovery.

Why didn't all of those tested show this same continuing improvement? Why did some decline, yet others continued to grow? After sifting through various possibilities, Schaie concludes that persons with "flexible personality styles" are more likely to continue to perform at high ability levels as they age. Intellectual competence so reflects the way we have lived our lives that, as Schaie says, ". . . it is typically only by age 81 that one can show that the average older person will fall below the middle range of performance for young adults."[6]

Schaie pinpoints, in addition to a flexible personality style, two other conditions for continuing high mental abilities: first, a favorable, less stressful personal situation; and second, freedom from arthritis and cardiovascular disease. Finally, Schaie roundly confirmed the general theses of this book when he said, "I find myself concluding that the use-it-or-lose it principle applies not only to the maintenance of muscular flexibility, but to the maintenance of flexible lifestyles and a related high level of intellectual performance as well."[7]

Chapter 12

Expectation: The Role of Mental Attitude

"Expectation" is one of the most important words in the English language. Its importance has to do with the most inescapable feature of human existence: time.

We live in time, which is to say we live with constant change: This minute gives way to the next; this day gives way to the next; and this year gives way to the next. Living and aging are identical events, because humans live in time, their lives changing from present time to future time. At the cutting edge of that change is expectation.

Expectation is what carries us from the present into the future. As such, it is like the prow of a vessel nosing its way forward. The direction in which the prow is pointed determines the direction the vessel will go. The prow leads the movement of the vessel. If the prow points up, the vessel will follow in the same direction: upward. If the prow points down, the vessel will go downward. The course of our life follows our expectations in the same way that a vessel follows the direction of its prow.

The expression, "a self-fulfilling prophecy," means that what we expect will happen usually turns out to be what actually happens. Expectation is not only a prediction of the future, it also directly contributes to making it happen. This proactive role which expectation plays is crucial to our well-being. Consider the placebo effect. This curious word is Latin. It means "I shall please," and it was taken from the liturgy of the Catholic Church, in which the priest said, "I shall please the lord . . ." Later, it came to be applied more generally to any attempt to flatter or please another person. By the nineteenth century it was being used by physicians to refer to any ineffective substance given as "medicine," not to cure, but merely to please, the patient. Soon, however, physicians began to notice an odd thing. These substances, which were not supposed to have any effect, actually succeeded if the physician cajoled the patient into believing it would. If the patient expected that the sugar pill would help, it did. This is the placebo effect.

Those in the medical profession are apt to think that their techniques are all that patients need. But the placebo effect contradicts this. F. J. Evans conducted a series of carefully controlled studies in pain reduction, which compared the effects of morphine to the effects of a "worthless" placebo pill. The findings were startling: The placebo was 56 percent as effective as a dose of morphine.[1] What could cause such a powerful analgesic effect? Only one thing: expectation.

Almost the same results were obtained in comparing placebo effects with those of aspirin (54 percent), codeine (56 percent), and Darvon (45 percent). It was extraordinary to learn that the placebo effect was constant. No matter what the analgesic drug, the effectiveness of the placebo was always proportional.

But, as the information poured in, physicians learned that the placebo effect was not at all limited to pain reduction; it was found in studies of adrenal gland secretion, angina, asthma, blood cell counts, blood pressure, cancer, the common cold, the cough reflex, diabetes, emesis, fever, gastric secretion and motility, headache, insomnia, multiple sclerosis, oral contraceptives, parkinsonism, pupil dilation and constriction, respiration, rheumatoid arthritis, seasickness, ulcers, vaccines, vasomotor function, and warts.[2] Such a list constitutes a massive confirmation of the somatic viewpoint—that human consciousness is an integral part of the human body's self-regulation.

The influence expectation has on people is so consistent and widespread that the pharmaceutical industry automatically takes it into consideration when it does its drug testing. In the lab, there is a "double-blind" arrangement. Neither the testers nor the subjects know which is the real drug and which is the placebo. Thus, Evans concludes: "The placebo should be considered a potent therapeutic intervention in its own right, an active agent whose positive or negative effects can be independently evaluated and whose mode of action is worthy of independent investigation."[3]

Not only are placebo effects seen in the area of pharmacology, they even compete with surgery. H. Beecher's classic medical study, "Surgery as a Placebo,"[4] recounts how placeboic surgery was used to reduce the pain of angina pectoris. The usual surgery involves making a skin incision and tying off the mammary artery. But some surgeons were skeptical, so they divided up into two teams, one making the incision and performing the mammary-artery ligation and the other simply making an incision and doing nothing else. The results were remarkable. The team making the incision and doing nothing else reported that 100 percent of their patients showed an increased ability to exercise and a reduced need for the painkiller, nitroglycerine. This same group of patients, when examined six weeks later, then six months later, still showed these same remarkable improvements. The other group showed only 76 percent improvements.

Placebo effects are evident also in the practice of biofeedback and in psychotherapy. Anxiety, edema, tachycardia, vasoconstriction, phobias, and depressions have all been relieved through the application of placebos. Clearly expectation is a factor in all human pathologies.

Because the placebo is so prevalent in clinical medicine, a science called psychoneuroimmunology has emerged. This promising research area presumes something that not too long ago was deemed impossible: that the immune system is not isolated in its functions, but has a working relation with the central nervous system. In addition, emotions, attitudes, and other conscious states trigger certain neurotransmittors which, in turn, affect the immune system—hence, the young science's name, psychoneuroimmunology.

The working thesis of psychoneuroimmunology is that a state of consciousness, such as an expectation, can cause changes in both the central nervous system and the immune system. This is essentially the somatic viewpoint: that the attitudes and beliefs we have about our bodies and our health vitally affect the ongoing state of our bodies and our health. If we expect our bodies to be resilient and healthy, then they will tend to remain so. On the other hand, expectation may be predicated on the myth of aging; that is, a belief in inevitable structural breakdown and functional loss. In this case, breakdown and loss will eventually occur. The prophecy becomes self-fulfilling: What we expect to happen does happen.

If we are at a certain age and feel within our bodies certain discomforts, how we interpret them becomes crucial. If we take them as a sign of serious disease and breakdown expected at this age in life, then we are accepting and giving in to a presumed fatality. To anticipate pathology is, functionally, tantamount to intending it. This unleashes dangerous reactions in the brain and in the immune system, dangerous because apparently the mere feeling of "giving in" to an ailment immobilizes our self-healing capacities.

If we habitually cringe in response to bodily discomforts, expecting the worst, we are chronically reinforcing this discomfort as a permanent condition, which then becomes resistant to improvement. Professor Ian Wickramasekera is a medical research scientist. In his general analysis of the placebo as a conditioned response, he says the following about this aspect of negative expectation:

> This analysis may be particularly relevant to chronic diseases and functional disorders such as low back pain, diabetes, cardiovascular disorders, musculoskeletal disorders, and cancer, in which the long-term and intermittent reinforcements of the unconditioned disease process, injury, or dysfunction *increase the probability of negative conditioned effects that sustain the disorder.* In such cases, the chronic intermittent activation of the disease mechanisms by unconditioned physiochemical causes may lead to *increasingly strong aversive anticipatory responses that inhibit the motor system even when the unconditioned stimulus is inactive.* It is a well-established fact that *intermittent reinforcement* by unconditioned stimuli *will make a maladaptive response maximally resistant to improvement.*[5]

This statement makes it clear that the myth of aging is not merely a belief about the diseases of aging; it can also be an active cause of these diseases. Thus, by responding to bodily discomforts with intelligent awareness and positive countermeasures, we can directly prevent such a "disease process, injury, or dysfunction" from becoming a permanent condition.

In brief, if we are intelligently aware of our bodies, and if we use positive countermeasures such as Somatic Exercises to improve our bodily self-regulation, the presumed "inevitable effects of aging" will, by and large, not occur.

Interlude: Learning to Drink from the Well

The word "age" means, quite simply, "a period of existence." It is one of the more fascinating words in the English language, because it is significantly more complex than it sounds. First of all, it has a curious etymology. Its Latin root is *aetus.* Its form, *aticus,* meaning "belonging to" or "proper to," was commonly used as a termination to many words: for example, *silvaticus,* "of the wood" *(silva),* and *viaticus,* "of the way" *(via).* Later, *aticus* evolved into the French suffix, *age,* and *silvaticus* passed into English as "savage" and *viaticus* as "voyage." Age became a common suffix in many English words: language, village, marriage, postage, and so on.

Moreover, even though "age" means simply "a period of existence," it refers more broadly to that which *characterizes* a period of existence. It is particularly interesting when it becomes a verb—to age—for then it means "to grow old." What, we should ask, does it mean "to grow old"? "Old," in its Latin root, *alo,* and in its ancient Germanic form, *alt,* means—quite surprisingly—"to nourish" and "to bring up." More generally, *alo* means to strengthen, increase, and advance. It means to become taller and to become deeper. In its root meaning, then, "to age," and to get older, means "to grow up." In view of the etymology of "old," it is fascinating to note that "growing old" has come to mean exactly the opposite of the original meaning of "old": that is, "old" has come to mean worn out, deteriorated, decayed, dilapidated, and no longer useful.

Thus, in plumbing the meaning of the simple but curious word, "age," we come upon a fundamental ambiguity: "To age" means either to grow, increase, and become both taller and deeper or to decrease, decay, wear out, and become decrepit and discarded.

It is most provocative that a word as basic to human life as "aging" can mean either of two opposite possibilities: growth or degeneration. It suggests that what is characteristic to the period of existence of a human's lifetime is neither programmed nor predictable. It implies that the direction of human life is not fixed but open.

This fundamental ambiguity reflects an abiding human insight into the ambiguity of aging: A human life can unfold in the direction of growth and increasing strength, or it can just as well unfold in the direction of decay and steady degeneration.

From the layered depths of our language arises the tantalizing suggestion that aging might mean growth rather than decay. This linguistic implication is tightly interlaced with the etymological roots of "aging," almost like the expression of a "collective unconscious" of our race—a collective insight into the authentic possibilities of human life. This insight has for millennia lain glowing within the heart of our language, awaiting full discovery and confirmation.

We now know enough about expectation and the way it mobilizes our bodies to realize that it is crucial, when we think of aging as a process, to distinguish between the two opposite meanings of "to age"—that is, to grow, or to decay. If we think of the coming years of our life as a continuing process of advancement and strengthening, it is more than likely we shall experience just that. And it is just as likely that a constant, daily expectation of wearing out and becoming decrepit will be a self-fulfilling prophecy.

Expectation is the leading edge of a belief system, and it has the curious feature of being self-justifying. As a leading edge, it predetermines our future. It programs what is to come, so that 60 years later one human smiles and affirms the progress of his life, saying, "This is just what I expected"; but another, who also says, "This is just what I expected," grimaces at his self-predicted decrepitude. Both got what they expected. They could not imagine it happening any other way.

Time is the currency spent by life, so we cannot wait for 60 years, wondering indecisively what to expect. Sixty years later will be too late.

We see in this situation an extraordinary truth about human life: Whether we will grow or degenerate during the course of our lives is a question not of known fact but of expected possibility. Time, as the currency of life, is always futurity; it is not yet spent. How we expect it to be spent predetermines the plan for its expenditure. Once we realize that the investment we make in our lives is the same as any other investment, we may adopt a very different attitude about what possibilities we expect for our future years.

I do not think it improper to say that what we invest in life determines how much we get out of it. It is a question of whether we think that our lives are at least as important an investment as, for example, real estate or stocks. It is my observation that many humans do not value their personal bodily future as highly as they value the future of their material possessions. Undoubtedly, they get their reward, which is "what they expected." To expand slightly a famous comment on the situation: "For what shall it profit a man, if he shall gain the whole world, and lose his own soul—and body?"

But life need not unfold in this way. We now know enough about expectation and the way it mobilizes our bodies to willingly choose the expectation that our conjoint souls and bodies—our "somas"—will "increase," "advance," become "deeper and taller"—partly because they are "nourished" and "brought up" with this happy expectation.

The human who knows that his or her being is growing is a human who usually has the strength and endurance to prevail over the defeats and stresses and traumas that occur in each and every life. Such a person knows that the inevitable pains and dysfunctions occurring in the body are not "inevitable signs of degeneration," but typical adjustments that all bodies go through in regulating and readapting themselves for the future.

A human who knows aging to be a process of ongoing growth is a human who has the ongoing power to overcome ailments, surmount malaise, and triumph over the worst of defeats. Not to countenance defeat, not to accept failure, not to give up, is to drink from the well of life's richest nourishment: the wisdom that, in its depth, life is ever redemptive and rejuvenating.

A Pride in Age

One effect of the myth of aging is that is induces us to despise old age and adulate youth. Worshiping youth is the inverse side of hating advancing age. It is regrettable that this attitude seems to have become steadily more popular, almost directly counter to the recent sudden expansion of our elderly population.

Is it that there are more people now who see their advancing years as something ominous and catastrophic? And is it that they hopelessly yearn for a state of youth that can never again be? Is this yearning so desperate that they will do anything to have at least the semblance of youth, masking the shameful signs of age so that, at least externally, they seem to give lie to the inescapable fact of aging skin and hair?

Let me say this as emphatically as possible: To despise the fact of aging is not only to despise life but to betray a pitiful ignorance of the nature of life.

Youth is not a state to be preserved but a state to be transcended. Youth has strength, but it does not have skill, which, in the long run, is the most potent strength. Youth has speed, but it does not have efficiency, which, in the long run, is the only effective way of attaining goals. Youth is quick, but it is not deliberate, and deliberation is the only way to make correct decisions. Youth has energy and intelligence, but it does not have the judgment necessary to make the best use of that energy and intelligence. Measured judgment in the end, is the only guarantor of intelligent behavior. Youth has the beauty of genetic endowment, but it does not have the beauty of real achievement. Youth has the glow of promise, but it does not have the radiance of accomplishment. Youth is a time of seeding and cultivation, but it is not a time of fruiting and harvest. Youth is a state of ignorance and innocence, but it is not a state of knowledge and wisdom. Youth is a state of emptiness awaiting fullness, a state of possibility awaiting actualization, a state of beginning awaiting transcendence.

In short, youth is a state to be put behind us as we grow taller and deeper and fuller. Unless we understand that life and aging are a process of growth and progress, we will never know the first principles of living. Nor will we understand what youth is all about: an explosive yearning to grow taller and deeper and fuller and to transcend oneself. It is by losing this yearning that we forget the first principles of living and begin to worship a false and superficial image of youthfulness.

The human species, possessed with a brain whose genius is unlimited learning and adaptation, is a species that is genetically designed to age by growing. Not to expect to grow is to misunderstand what it means to be human. Not to do so is to fail in the God-given task of living a fully human life. To expect the opposite is, in effect, to sin against life and its biological promise.

As we move toward a new moment in history when one-quarter of the population will be 65 years or older, we must remind and reeducate ourselves to the full possibilities contained in the entire human life span. In our worship of youth, and in our frantic scramble to falsify our age, we have blindly ignored a growing number of discoveries that can make life and aging a continuing process of growth, achievement, satisfaction, and pleasure. My primary concern is to present scientific and practical information about discoveries that can free us from the fear of aging. Fear of aging is a product of ignorance, and this ignorance is no longer defensible, any more than the myth of aging is defensible. The laboratory and clinical research reviewed earlier and the Somatic Exercises that follow in Part 3 are the instruments with which we can begin to reverse our traditional superstitions about aging. This reversal can come about, not with more doctors, more hospitals, and more nursing homes, but with more self-conscious, self-regulating, individuals who have educated themselves in the ways of controlling the process of their own lives.

During this epochal upward shift in population, it is not more "hard" technologies we need. It is new "soft" technologies, such as those we have discussed. The soft technologies are the somatic technologies that teach us internal control of our own physiological and psychological lives. The Somatic Exercises—which are not to be read with the "mind" but learned through both the body and the mind—are a soft technology.

This is an age of "software," where the "programs" for the machines are more significant than the machines themselves. Computers are totally useless without their programs. It is the right program in the right computer language that unlocks the magic of the cybernetic process. In exactly the same manner, it is the right method and the right understanding of somatic practice that is the key for unlocking the magic of the human central nervous system, and of keeping it unlocked during the whole of one's life.

Not only is it possible to overcome and avoid the effects of sensory-motor amnesia, it is also possible to have a body and a life that are lasting sources of productivity and satisfaction and pride. I believe that, more than anything else, it is pride in age that must be restored to our lives—to be happy with aging, to savor its promise and to enjoy its unfolding. Every human being should school himself and herself in looking forward to aging as a promise to be fulfilled. If we are to learn anything from youth, it is just this—for the burning essence of youthfulness is to look forward to aging as a beckoning promise of happiness and fulfillment.

This is the attitude of youth that we must keep from birth through maturity and till death, for it is an attitude of positive expectation: to expect the best of our lives and to have the basic somatic skills to guarantee this expectation. Such an attitude and such skills can make for a very different elderly population. It is my conviction that the most extraordinary gerontological event will not be the age shift in the population but the shift in attitude and accomplishment of the elderly.

I envisage a totally practicable possibility of an emerging elderly population with the skills, efficiency, deliberation, judicious use of energy, measured judgment, and real abilities of achievement and accomplishment to become the most significant portion of the population. Even the briefest reflection tells us that this is obvious: that the most experienced, skilled, and learned portion of our population should be the source of our most reliable leadership and most impressive abilities. And it is my contention that, with the means of avoiding the age-old plague of sensory-motor amnesia, and with a positive expectation that creates pride in age, this event has every likelihood of coming about. The enormous capacity of the human brain almost guarantees that such a shift in the quality of mature human life can occur, once humans master the personal, adaptive skills of controlling the internal processes of their lives.

To say that aging is an adventure is the same as saying that life is an adventure. Indeed, each individual life is the greatest adventure. Together, they are part of the larger adventure, a life of community evolving on a blue and green planet as it spins its course through a measureless universe. The human race is changing. At the present moment, this change is accelerating, and is charged with the thrill of danger and promise. That's what it feels like when the currents of futurity gather momentum and move us forward headlong into the future.

We must make our way through this great time of change, expecting that it will be good, and intending that it will be good. We must make our future the way we want it to be. That is what human freedom is for. And, in the process, we may discover that the myth of aging has been replaced by another, brighter myth. If it is true that, in the deepest reaches of the human heart, we all live according to myths, we may find that, from the ashes of the old myth, a new myth of aging is arising: that life is a continuous process of growth and expansion.

PART 3

The Somatic
Exercise Program

I designed these Somatic Exercises specifically to reduce the effects of sensory-motor amnesia that normally occur by middle age. They are based on the ingenious work of Dr. Moshe Feldenkrais, an Israeli scientist. In 1975, I sponsored and directed the first Feldenkrais training course in the United States. Since that time, his revolutionary method of body reeducation has been taught worldwide.

This program consists not of physical exercises but of Somatic Exercises; it offers specific procedures for making changes in the sensory-motor areas of the brain in order to maintain internal control of the muscle system. Because you are exercising your brain as well as your body, it is important to practice each movement pattern with your maximum conscious attention.

The program is progressive and gradual, centering on the areas of the body where SMA occurs. The first four Somatic Exercises train you in sensitivity and control of the muscles in the middle of your body, at its center of gravity. The next two deal with the periphery of your body: namely, your legs, arms, and neck. The final two exercises focus on two major functions of your body: breathing and walking, both of which are typically limited by SMA.

Chapter 13

How to Give Yourself the Maximum Benefit of Somatic Exercises

The most important thing for you to remember is that Somatic Exercises change your muscular system by changing your central nervous system. If you do not remember this important fact, their effectiveness will be diminished for you.

You will receive the maximum benefit from the eight movement patterns that make up the Somatic Exercises if you do the following:

1. *Learn the nature of sensory-motor amnesia, how it occurs in your brain, and where it occurs in your body, by reading and reviewing Part 2.* Understanding your brain and body and how they are affected by stress and trauma is essential for the benefits of Somatic Exercises to last. For most people, the initial effect of these movement patterns "feels like" magic as their bodies relax and regain their suppleness. But the "real" magic comes from learning how to maintain your suppleness and how to continue developing it.

As your internal sensitivity and control grow, look back from time to time at the information contained in different sections of *Somatics.* You will discover that certain passages and chapters take on more and more meaning as you come to understand your body better. And the more you understand about your body, the more you can discover about yourself through these exercises.

2. *While doing the Somatic Exercises, your primary task is to focus your attention on the internal sensations of movement.* These movement patterns highlight those areas of the body most commonly affected by sensory-motor amnesia. As you perform the exercises, concentrate on developing a careful sensory awareness of the movements in these body areas as a direct way to maintain control over them.

To this end, the instructions on performing each individual movement are immediately followed by instructions for sensing each one. In this way, you will know what to look for in the feelings of sensory feedback that these movement patterns evoke.

3. Ideally, you should do your Somatic Exercises while lying on a rug or mat, wearing loose clothing, and being away from all distractions. A rug or mat allows comfort while providing a firm support for your body. This allows you to be more precise in performing the movement and more precise in perceiving it. People whose movement or strength is extremely limited may do their Somatic Exercises in bed. The firmer their mattresses, the more effective the exercises will be, and they should move to a rug or mat as soon as possible.

The object of Somatic Exercises is to loosen your body from constricted muscles, so it makes no sense to wear constricting clothing while you do them. On the other hand, there's no need for athletic gear. You're not supposed to work up a sweat doing Somatic Exercises.

Finally, you should avoid areas of your home where you will be interrupted or distracted. You will need to concentrate on the movement patterns and how they feel inside your body. Therefore, being in a room where a television is on, or even where music is playing, will interfere with your learning. You might think that a mirror will help you position your body correctly, but actually, it might mislead you. It is more important to perceive the movements through your sensory-motor system than through your eyes.

One way to preserve your concentration is to have the instructions for your Somatic Exercises read aloud to you as you do them, so that you do not have to stop to read each one. If you have a tape recorder, record the lessons on a tape at the right speed so that they are always handy.

4. Always move slowly. Moving slowly, you give your brain the chance to notice all that is happening in your body as you move. Slow-motion films are essential in sports training because they allow athletes to study the details of a movement or play. The same goes for focusing attention on the internal sensations of your own movements: The slower you go, the more you perceive.

Furthermore, although you will experience bodily changes almost from the beginning of the first exercise, do not go on to the next until your mind is completely clear about what you are doing and until you can do it with ease and comfort. It is best to repeat each lesson at least once before going to the next. Somatic Exercises are programmed at progressive levels, so that successful learning depends on having mastered the movements at the previous levels. In this way your mastery is solid, and can become part of your regular pattern of movements.

5. Always move gently and with the least possible effort. This, again, is so that your brain can receive precise and uncluttered sensory feedback from the exercises. When you experience excessive effort and strain—as is usually the case in doing calisthenics—then your brain is cluttered by sensory feedback that is irrelevant to what you are relearning to control. It is better for you to feel that you are doing "too little" than to risk doing too much and undermining the somatic learning process.

6. Do not force any movement.   Somatic Exercises help you maintain sensitivity and control, but, until your brain learns how to move your muscles, no amount of force and effort will release the involuntary contractions in your body. Pushing against your muscles is from the old tradition of physical training, which always fails to release the hold of sensory-motor amnesia. If you attempt to voluntarily force a muscle that is involuntarily contracted, you will cause an equal and opposite resistance of that muscle. It will contract even tighter, finally to the point of spasm.

Remember: If you want to untie a knot, you must look at the cord carefully and then gently undo the tangle. Yanking on the cord will only make the knot tighter.

7. Somatic Exercises are not painful.   The movement patterns of these exercises are the normal movements of the musculoskeletal system. If you perform them slowly and gently, they are completely harmless. Hurting yourself while exercising is unnecessary, harmful, and, of course, no fun at all.

Often people with tight, sore muscles make matters worse by protectively tightening their muscles even further so as to avoid moving them at all. Remember that life is movement, and no one can avoid moving. The act of breathing, for example, automatically brings a constantly alternating pressure on your spine. Because movement is unavoidable, we should be sure to move in directions that are, anatomically and neurologically, the least harmful—that is how Somatic Exercises are designed.

People who are already suffering from sensory-motor amnesia, especially those with severely contracted lower back muscles, will sometimes feel soreness when these muscles first begin to lengthen. This is to be expected; and once their muscles lengthen, the soreness will disappear. Even very painful lower back muscles become comfortable after about three days of Somatic Exercises, once they have relaxed to their natural length and blood has circulated through the muscle fibers. Thus, if you feel some pain doing the exercises, move gently and slowly, never forcing your movements, and keep in mind that this is the normal direction of movement that you are trying to reestablish.

There are always unusual situations where normal musculoskeletal movement patterns are impossible because of an observable obstacle. In such cases, you should seek medical advice and follow it. Physicians usually agree that Somatic Exercises are anatomically harmless when done properly.

8. Be persistent, patient, and positive.   Somatic Exercises change your body by teaching your brain. Your learning grows steadily and solidly. You must be persistent—determined in your practice of these movement patterns. You must be patient—looking not for a "quick fix" on your body, but for a genuine, lasting change in your comfort, range of movement, posture, and general functioning. Most importantly, you must be positive in your expectations, envisaging and aiming for the improvement you know your somatic system is capable of.

Interlude: **The Daily "Cat Stretch"**

After you have mastered bodily control, you will arrive at a new stage of your Somatic Exercises: *maintenance of your sensory-motor control.* You must preserve what you have learned as a normal and permanent aspect of your bodily habits without any loss or erosion due to the daily stresses to which you may be subjected.

While the learning stage requires patient attention, the maintenance stage requires only a short time each day to reinforce what you have learned. All that is required is a brief repetition of your basic movement patterns, to remind the sensory-motor tracts of your brain how to do them. Therefore, your Daily "Cat Stretch" consists of the most important movements from your Somatic Exercises.

I am often asked, "How long must I continue doing these maintenance movements?" My reply is, "How many years must a cat continue to stretch after it wakes up?" The answer for cats is the same as for humans: at least once a day, preferably just after waking up.

Because a cat's muscles and connective tissue shorten while it sleeps, after waking up it stretches them back to their previous length. Most animals stretch when they awaken in order to maintain their full range of muscular control. Our muscles and brains are no different in this respect from those of other animals. Hence, your maintenance movements are not to be thought of as "exercises" any more than a cat thinks of them as such—they are the natural way of preparing your body to feel good throughout the day.

Doing your Daily "Cat Stretch" for five minutes each day upon awakening is sufficient to reinforce what your brain has learned so that you will never suffer sensory-motor amnesia. Many people prefer to do the same routine for five minutes at night just before retiring. That way they go to sleep with the movement patterns freshly reinforced in their brains, and it helps them sleep more soundly. If your day has been stressful, making your muscles tight and fatigued, you will find that a "Cat Stretch" automatically relieves your tension.

If you suffer a traumatic event—an injury, surgery, or a tragic personal experience—it is advisable to return to the basic program of Somatic Exercises. Carefully go through each lesson, one by one, to be sure you overcome any involuntary constrictions caused by your trauma. Then return to your "Cat Stretch" each day.

The Daily "Cat Stretch"

Like all Somatic Exercises, these maintenance movements should be done slowly, gently, and with maximum awareness. Do them in an easygoing, catlike manner so that they give you pleasure.

1. Lying on your back, arch and flatten your lower back, inhaling while going up and exhaling while going down. Repeat five times over thirty seconds. *Lesson One: 1.B.*

2. Lying on your back with both hands interlaced behind your head, lift your head while exhaling and flattening your back. Lower your head while inhaling and arching your back. Repeat five times over thirty seconds. *Lesson One: 5.A.*

3. Lying on your stomach with your left cheek on the back of your right hand, lift your head, hand, and right elbow while simultaneously lifting your left leg. Do this two times, then do the same for the other side of your body. Inhale slowly while lifting; exhale slowly while coming down. This will take about thirty seconds. *Lesson One: 2.E and 3.E.*

4. Lying on your back with your left knee held by your left hand, lift your head and right elbow to your left knee while exhaling and flattening your back. As your head comes down, inhale, arching your back up. Repeat three times. Do the same for the other side of your body three times. This will take about sixty seconds. *Lesson Two: 3.A and 4.A.*

5. Lying on your back, roll your arms in opposite directions on the floor, alternately dropping your knees each time to the side of the arm rolling down the floor. Turn your head in the direction opposite your knees to make a full spinal twist. Move slowly and lazily, so as to enjoy the stretch. Repeat six times over thirty seconds. *Lesson Four: 8.A.*

6. Lying on your back, twist your right foot, leg, and hip in and out five times, being sure to lift and arch each side of your back alternately without lifting your shoulders. Do the same with your left side. Move both legs simultaneously in alternating bow-legged/knock-kneed positions five times, then together in skiing motions five times. This will take about sixty seconds. *Lesson Five: 3.A, 6.A, 7.A, and 7.B.*

7. Sitting with your right hand on your left shoulder and with both knees bent and facing left, rotate your trunk to the left three times. Holding your trunk motionless at full left turn, turn your head to the right and back three times. Turn both your head and your trunk in alternate directions three times for the full spinal twist. Still holding your trunk to the left, lift your face to the ceiling while dropping your eyes to the floor and *vice versa* three times. Do the same for the other side of your body. This will take about sixty seconds. *Lesson Six: 1.A and 1.B for both sides; 3.A for both sides; and 4.A and 4.B for both sides.*

Chapter 14

The Somatic Exercises[1]

LESSON 1
Controlling the Extensor Muscles of the Back

The first movement pattern deals with the muscles of the back, which are activated by the Green Light reflex. When this reflex becomes habituated, it causes the most common ailment in industrialized societies: lower back pain.

Because you are just beginning to explore this area of frequent soreness and aching, start out with small, cautious movements that are done slowly and attentively. At the end, repeat the lesson one more time to be certain that you understand the movement patterns and that you can do them with awareness and comfort.

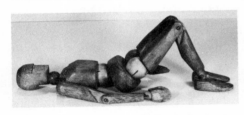

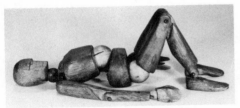

1. POSITION
Lie on back, knees bent, and feet near to buttocks.

A. MOVEMENT
Press pelvis down against the floor several times, then begin pressing the tailbone down more firmly than the rest of the pelvis. This will make the lower back arch up at the belt line.

SENSING
Slide one hand under the small of the back to feel how the muscles contract on both sides of your spine as you arch.

B. MOVEMENT
Now inhale as you arch the lower back and exhale as you flatten the

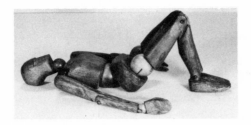

lower back down toward the floor. Gradually increase the range of this movement by pressing the tailbone down more firmly to lift the lower back higher, and then by pressing the lower back down more firmly, which slightly lifts the tailbone. (Do this movement slowly and gently about *20 times*.)

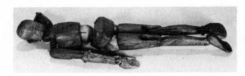

2. POSITION
Turn over onto your stomach, placing your left cheek down on the back of your right hand with the left hand lying alongside your body.

A. MOVEMENT
Slowly lift up the right elbow *3 times*.

SENSING
Try to feel which muscles in the shoulder are contracting.

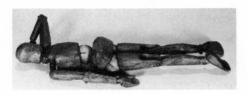

B. MOVEMENT
Slowly lift head to look over right shoulder *3 times*.

SENSING
Notice the contraction of muscles from the shoulder down the right side of the spine to the pelvis.

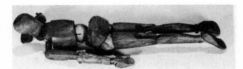

C. MOVEMENT
Simultaneously lift elbow, hand, and head to look over right shoulder *3 times*.

SENSING
Notice how the contraction has now extended through the shoulder girdle down the spine into the left buttocks, which contracts as if to lift the left leg.

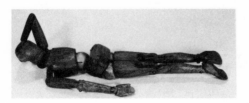

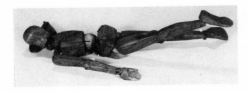

D. MOVEMENT
Now reverse this movement by lifting the left leg a few inches from the floor *3 times.*

SENSING
Notice how your brain balances the weight of the left leg by automatically contracting the muscles of both the right spine and shoulder.

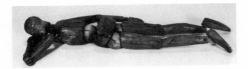

E. MOVEMENT
Do both movements simultaneously: Slowly inhale, lifting both the left leg and the right hand-elbow and head *3 times.*

---

3. POSITION
Now turn your head to the left, placing the right cheek on back of the left hand with the right hand lying alongside your body.

MOVEMENT
Same as above, i.e.,

A. Lift left elbow *3 times.*

B. Lift head to look over shoulder *3 times.*

C. Lift head, hand, and shoulder to look over left shoulder *3 times.*

D. Lift the right leg a few inches from the floor *3 times.*

E. Do both movements simultaneously: Slowly inhale, lifting both the right leg and the left hand-elbow and head *3 times.*

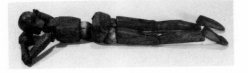

4. POSITION
Put left hand on back of right hand, placing center of forehead on back of left hand.

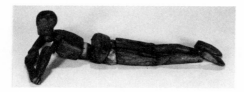

A. MOVEMENT
Inhale and slowly lift head and eyes up toward ceiling *3 times.*

SENSING
Feel how the muscles contract along both sides of the spine down into the buttocks. You are feeling the classic swaybacked posture with belly projected forward and head pulled backward that most adults mistakenly take to be "straight." This is the distorted Green Light reflex which causes most adults to have chronic back pain.

During the next five movements, notice the different areas of contraction in the neck, shoulder, back, buttocks, and hamstring muscles of the legs.

MOVEMENTS

B. Inhale, lifting up right leg a few inches, then lowering it as you exhale. *3 times.*

C. Inhale, lifting up left leg a few inches, then lowering it as you exhale. *3 times.*

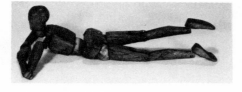

D. Inhale, lifting right leg and head simultaneously, then lowering them as you exhale. *3 times.*

E. Inhale, lifting left leg and head simultaneously, then lowering them as you exhale. *3 times.*

F. Inhale, *just slightly* lifting both legs and head *one time only.*

5. POSITION
Roll over onto your back again, knees bent, and feet near to buttocks. Interlace the fingers of both

hands and place them beneath back of head.

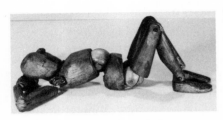

A. MOVEMENT

Inhale, arching your lower back (remember that when you do this the tailbone presses downward as the beltline rises); then exhale, flattening the lower back down toward the floor *as you lift your head. Repeat 6 times.*

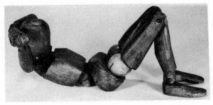

B. MOVEMENT

Relax now, stretching out hands and legs on the floor.

SENSING

Try to sense how your back feels as you lie in this relaxed position. Sense it from inside your body, then slip your hand flat under the lower back to feel whether the lower back is lying flatter on the floor.

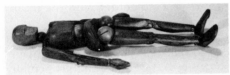

The Daily "Cat Stretch"

Already, you have learned four parts of the Daily "Cat Stretch," that you will be doing later as part of your maintenance routine. Please note that the movements you did in 1.B. and in 5.A. are the first two parts of the "Cat Stretch." These are followed by the movements of 2.E. and 3.E.

LESSON 2
Controlling the Flexor Muscles of the Stomach

This lesson teaches the rudiments of controlling the Red Light reflex, which flexes the muscles in the front of the body. Learning to control these muscles goes hand in hand with controlling their opposite muscle group: the extensor muscles of the back.

The flexor muscles pull in the opposite direction of the extensor muscles—one group is the agonist, and the other group is the antagonist. When they both pull at the same time, they squeeze the entire trunk in what has been called the Dark Vise—a condition directly related to shallow breathing and to distortion of heartbeat rhythm and blood pressure.

When you finish the movement of lifting the head toward the right knee while using the right hand, notice the difference in the way the right pelvis and the right shoulder blade lie against the rug. You will be asked throughout the lesson to be aware of your sensory feedback; this is just as important to learn as is improved muscle control. The sensory learning goes together with the motor learning.

At the end of the lesson, it is essential that you do the *Body Image Training*. It will reveal to you how sensory-motor amnesia creates a distorted body image: that is, even though you may believe you are sitting "straight," you may actually be sitting with a swayback. And when the back muscles have released enough to allow you to sit truly straight, you will, at first, feel as if you are slumped forward! At this point you will realize that, as of Lesson Two, your body is actually reorganizing its posture.

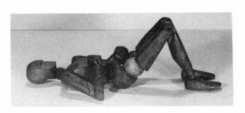

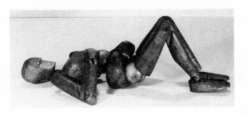

1. POSITION

Lie on back, knees bent, with feet near to buttocks. Place left hand on pubic bone and place right hand over lower half of chest. (N.B.: The abdominal muscle extends from the pubic bone to the mid-chest.)

A. MOVEMENT

Inhale, slowly lifting lower back as the pelvis rolls down to the tailbone; then exhale, flattening lower back. *Repeat 6 times.*

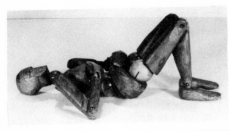

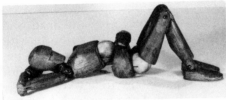

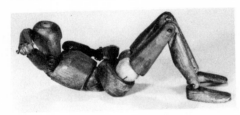

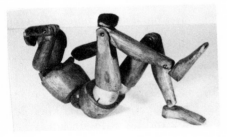

SENSING

Feel with your hands how the abdominal muscle contracts when you flatten the lower back. The emotions of fear and apprehension will also cause the abdominal muscle to contract—that is the Red Light reflex.

B. MOVEMENT

Place right hand beneath head, then inhale, arching back as you did before; then, exhale, contracting abdominal muscle to flatten lower back toward floor as you lift up head with right hand. *Repeat 6 times.*

SENSING

Use your left hand to notice how the abdominal muscle contracts even harder when you lift your head.

C. MOVEMENT

Now raise right knee and hold it in front with left hand. Continue same pattern as above, but now, as you exhale, flattening the back and lifting the head, *pull the right knee toward the elbow* and point the right elbow toward the right knee 6 *times.*

SENSING

Notice how the more you lower the back against the floor, the easier it is to bring the elbow to the knee. You are releasing the back muscles even farther now.

Stretch out arms and legs and relax, noticing how it feels down the trunk between the right shoulder and the right hip.

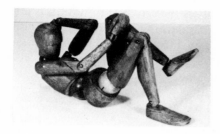

2. POSITION

On back, knees bent, with feet near to buttocks.

A. MOVEMENT

Begin, once again, the pattern of slowly inhaling, lifting the lower back, then exhaling, while flattening the lower back. . . .

B. MOVEMENT

Place left hand beneath head and hold front of left knee in the air with right hand. Now, as you lower the back, exhaling, simultaneously lift head and elbow to left knee, while pulling left knee toward left elbow. *6 times.*

SENSING

Notice that the more you lower the small of the back, the nearer the face and elbow will come to the knee. Your back muscles are beginning to release even more.

Stop, stretch out arms and legs to rest.

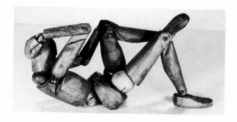

3. POSITION

On back with knees bent, place right hand beneath head. Then lift left knee and hold it with left hand.

A. MOVEMENT

Inhale, slowly lifting the lower back; then, as you exhale, flatten the back and lift the head and right elbow toward the left knee. Simultaneously, pull left knee toward right elbow and face. *6 times.*

SENSING

Notice how the head and elbow must point slightly to the left. Also feel how the more you round the back downward toward the floor, the nearer the elbow comes to the knee. Your back muscles are releasing still further and becoming more supple: i.e., you are remembering how to gain voluntary control again of the muscles of the back.

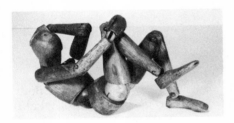

4. POSITION
Place left hand beneath head, then lift up the right knee and hold it with the right hand.

A. MOVEMENT
Inhale, arching lower back; then, as you exhale, lift the head and left elbow toward the right knee, while pulling the knee toward the left elbow and face. *6 times.*

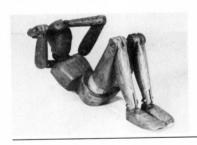

5. POSITION
Interlace both hands and place them beneath the back of the head.

A. MOVEMENT
Inhale, arching lower back, then exhale, flattening the back as you lift up the head. *3 times.*

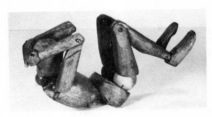

6. POSITION
Keep hands beneath head, lift up both knees, letting them balance over the stomach.

A. MOVEMENT
Inhale, arching up lower back; then exhale, flattening back as the hands lift the head and both elbows toward both knees. Try to bring the knees toward the elbows.

Stretch out legs with arms alongside body and rest.

SENSING

Notice how you feel inside your body from the middle of the chest down to the pubic bone and in the area between the legs. As you quietly inhale, allow your lower belly to rise freely with complete relaxation, so that your breathing becomes deep and full.

Body Image Training

After repeating Lesson Two and becoming more able to release and flatten the lower back, practice this same movement while you are sitting. If you have had chronic lower back pains for many years, you will have a swayback with very contracted muscles along each side of the lower spine.

If that has been your chronic condition, you will discover—through Body Image Training—how sensory-motor amnesia has caused you to forget what it means for the lower back to be relaxed and more vertical, with the weight resting on the vertebrae.

Because SMA creates a distorted body image, when your back is relaxed and flat, and when your head is directly over the center of gravity of your body, *you will feel too far forward, as if you were slumped.* Because you have held the back for so long in an unnatural (and uncomfortable!) position, it has come to feel "normal" being that way—even though you have had recurrent pains with the swayed back and its contraction of the lumbar muscles.

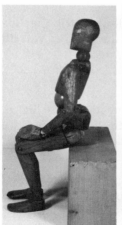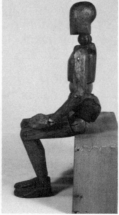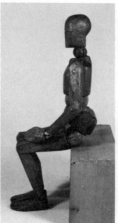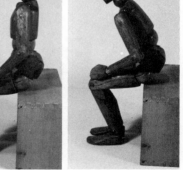

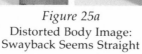

Figure 25a
Distorted Body Image:
Swayback Seems Straight

Figure 25b
Straight Back Seems "Slumped"

Hence, when your back now begins to relax and your upper trunk can come forward again to a natural, unstressed posture, notice how "abnormal" it feels at first. This is only a transient experience that will pass away within a week or so as the relaxed posture begins to feel normal.

It is essential that you deal directly with the distorted body image caused by SMA. Otherwise, learning how to release the chronically held muscles of the lower back will not, by itself, lead to a permanent change in your comfort and height or in the way you habitually sit.

I ask my clients to practice relaxing and flattening their lower back while sitting, with their eyes closed in a chair that is turned sideways to a mirror. When they internally sense that they have relaxed their backs, they will—while in a sitting posture—feel abnormally "slumped forward."

But then, when I ask them to open their eyes and look at their image in the mirror, they are astonished to discover that their back is both tall and vertical— and also that the belly is flat.

Please make use of this mirror technique. It is a simple and fascinating example of biofeedback.

When your internal sense of back position and your visual sense of back position finally adjust to one another, your way of sitting will be permanently changed. You will be able to sit for hours without soreness or fatigue, because your vertebrae will be a vertical column of support for the trunk—exactly as the mirror shows it to be. It is just a matter of getting used to a new body image.

And, in addition, you will be taller. Why? Because a straight line is longer than a curved line!

The Daily "Cat Stretch"
Please note that you have now learned two more parts of your Daily "Cat Stretch" routine: 3.A. and 4.A.

LESSON 3
Controlling the Muscles of the Waist

If you are short-waisted, these movement patterns will help make you visibly longer-waisted. If your trunk tends to tilt to one side, Lesson Three will bring you more toward verticality.

When you have finished the movements on the right side, be sensitive to the feeling of length that has come into this side. You may also notice that there is more movement in the waist when you inhale. You are cultivating greater somatic self-awareness, and this sensory ability allows you to be more capable of self-monitoring what is happening in your body.

1. POSITION
Lie on left side, knees folded on top of each other at right angles to the body. Extend left arm on floor, so that left ear can rest on it, like a cushion. Reach right hand over top of head, placing the palm of the right hand against left ear.

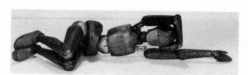

A. MOVEMENT
Inhale and, using right arm, very slowly lift the head into the air. Then exhale, letting the head slowly come back down. *3 times.*

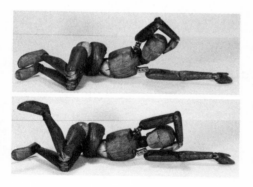

B. MOVEMENT
Inhale and very slowly lift up right lower leg and foot, rolling (but not lifting) right thigh. Then exhale, letting the foot slowly come back down. Pretend that you are lifting up the right hip to touch the right armpit. *3 times.*

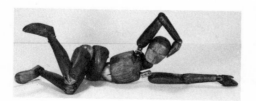

C. MOVEMENT
Inhale and very slowly lift *both* head and right foot in air. Then exhale, letting them both come down simultaneously. Pretend that you are lifting the right armpit to place over the right hip. *3 times.*

Lie on your back and rest one minute, with arms alongside body and feet slightly apart.

SENSING
As you rest, sense within your body how it feels in the mid-section. Can you notice any difference between the left and right sides?

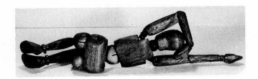

2. POSITION
Turn over onto right side with knees folded on top of each other at right angles to the body. Extend the right arm on the floor, so that the right ear can rest on it like a cushion. Reach left arm over top of head, placing the palm against the right ear.

A. MOVEMENT
Inhale and, using left arm, very slowly lift up head in the air as high as is comfortable. *3 times.* Does it go up more easily than the right side? Or less easily?

B. MOVEMENT
Inhale and very slowly lift left foot in the air as high as is comfortable. Let the thigh roll but do not lift it. Your left hip will contract and lift toward the left shoulder. Exhale, letting the foot come back down slowly. *3 times.*

C. MOVEMENT
Inhale and very slowly lift both head and left foot in air as high as is comfortable. Then exhale, letting them come back down slowly. Pretend that you are bringing the left hip up to fit into the hollow of the left armpit. *3 times.*

Turn over onto your back and rest, with the arms alongside body and the feet slightly apart.

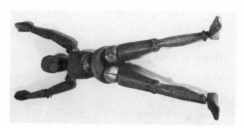

3. POSITION

Lying on your back, spread the feet a little wider than your hip joints. Then reach both arms straight above top of head against rug, spreading them wider than your shoulders. Your body will be like a large X lying on the rug with a straight line from the right arm down to the left leg and from the left arm down to the right leg.

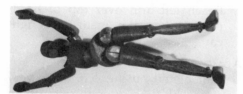

A. MOVEMENT

Slowly lengthen your right leg, stretching the heel down the floor.

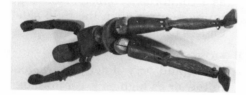

B. MOVEMENT

Relaxing the right leg, slowly lengthen your left arm above the head, sliding it along the rug. *Repeat this leg-arm movement 10 times.*

SENSING

Notice how your waist and rib cage on both sides change back and forth as you alternate stretching the right leg and left arm. Sense how your ability to reach depends on how freely you can move your waist and rib cage. You can see that a tight waist automatically restricts the movement of the leg in walking and the arm in reaching.

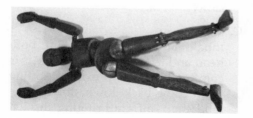

Stop and relax, so that you can compare the feelings in the right leg with the left and the feelings in the left arm and rib cage with that of the right.

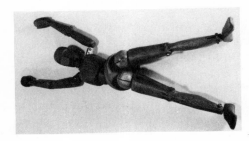

C. MOVEMENT

Slowly lengthen your left leg, stretching the heel down the floor.

D. MOVEMENT

Relaxing the left leg, slowly lengthen your right arm above the head, sliding it along the rug. *Repeat this leg-arm movement 10 times.*

Relax, and notice the greater feeling of similarity between the two sides.

E. MOVEMENT

Now put together these four movement directions in a rounded fashion: Stretch the left arm upward, then relax. Stretch the right leg downward, then relax. Stretch the left leg downward, then relax. Stretch the right arm upward, then relax. Stretch the left arm upward, then relax. Then the right leg, then left leg, then right arm, and so on. *Repeat this 4-point cycle 10 times.*

Stop and relax. You have now learned greater control and awareness of the muscles on the sides of the body, in addition to what you learned earlier about the back and front of the body. This prepares you for the next lesson, which involves using all of these muscles by rotating the body.

LESSON 4
Controlling the Muscles Involving Trunk Rotation

This Somatic Exercise takes full advantage of the growing sensitivity and control you have now attained in all three sections of the center of the body: the extensor muscles of the back, the flexor muscles of the abdomen, and the lateral muscles of the waist.

During the spiral twisting you will be doing in this lesson, your sensory-motor tracts can simultaneously experience the lengthening of all three muscle groups. Not only is the pelvis now beginning to move more freely, the entire spine and the rib cage are also. You will notice that, as you gain control of these areas, the body begins to reshape itself. As your chest, for example, is released from the depressing effect of the Red Light reflex, it lifts and expands.

At this stage of your neuromuscular training, you will begin to perceive how similar these movement patterns are to what a cat is doing when it stretches. You will notice the special pleasure that is sensed when the trunk stretches more freely.

This lesson ends with an easy-to-do resumé movement that involves inverse rotation of the arms and legs. Later on, you can include this in your Daily "Cat Stretch" routine. This movement is a full spiral twist, and it allows the trunk to stretch to its fullest length. Note that when the knees are dropped to one side and the head is turned to the opposite side, the entire body is twirled, exactly the way a washrag is spirally twisted when we wring it out, twisting one end clockwise and the other end counterclockwise. As you will learn in Lesson Eight, mastering this twist is essential to an easy stride in walking.

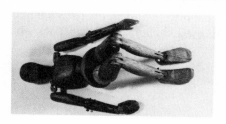

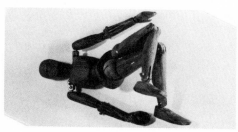

1. POSITION

Lie on your back with knees bent and feet near to buttocks.

A. MOVEMENT

Cross the left leg fully over the right leg. Inhale; then, as you exhale, allow the legs to tilt slowly down to the left as far as they will naturally fall. Then inhale and slowly lift them back to vertical; then exhale once again and allow the legs to slowly tilt back down to the left. *Repeat this movement 10 times.* Be sure that your right shoulder stays on the floor and does not lift as the legs drop left.

Stretch out your arms and legs and rest.

SENSING
Compare the feelings in the right hip and leg with those in the left. See if the right side of your chest feels more open than the left side.

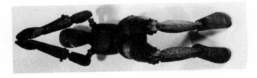

2. POSITION
Still lying on your back with knees bent, hold up both hands in the air, with the elbows straight and the palms pressed firmly together. The arms will be making the shape of a tall steeple. As you do the next movement, make certain that the elbows do not bend nor the palms slip. The knees will remain in the vertical position.

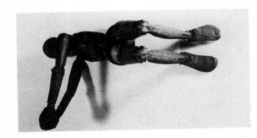

A. MOVEMENT
Inhale. Then, as you exhale, tilt the arms slowly to the right as far as is comfortable—also turning the eyes and head to the right. Then inhale and slowly lift the arms back to vertical; then exhale and tilt the arms down again to the right, *repeating this movement 5 times.*

Stretch out your arms and legs and rest.

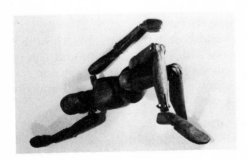

B. MOVEMENT
Now, once again, cross the left knee over the right (the arms remain down at your side) and exhale, allowing the legs to tilt down to the left. Roll your head to the right as you do this, and reach your arm up on the rug above the head, stretching as the knees drop. Inhale, lifting legs vertical, then exhale, dropping them down left again as you turn your head and stretch the arm, *repeating this 5 times.*

SENSING

Is it easier to drop the legs this second time? Do they seem to go farther? Think of how your upper body has been twisting to the right and your lower body to the left: Your body is forming a spiral, and your body is lengthening.

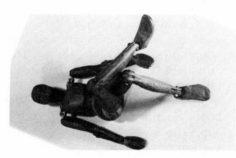

3. POSITION

On back with arms by side and knees bent, but this time cross the right leg over the left.

A. MOVEMENT

Exhale, letting the legs tilt slowly down to the right, then inhale, bringing them back to vertical. Then exhale again, letting the legs drop right again. Each time, roll the head left and stretch the left arm up on the rug over your head. *Repeat 10 times.*

SENSING

By turning the head, your neck vertebrae rotate to left, making it easier for the vertebrae and ribs in the middle of your trunk to space themselves and form the spiral twist.

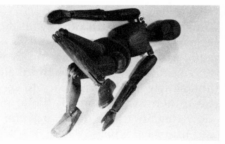

4. POSITION

Hold both hands straight up in the air, with elbows straight and palms pressed firmly together, making a steeple. The knees are bent and remain vertical.

A. MOVEMENT

Exhale, tilting the arms slowly to left. Inhale, bringing the arms back to vertical. Be sure the elbows and hands maintain their positions. *Repeat 5 times.*

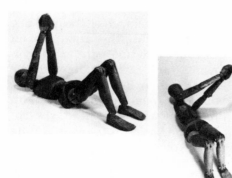

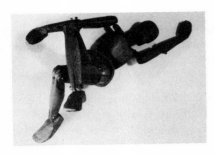

5. POSITION

Once again, cross the right leg over the left.

A. MOVEMENT

Exhale, tilting the legs slowly to the right, while rolling your head to the left and stretching the left arm upward on the rug. *5 times.*

SENSING

Notice the catlike grace of this stretching movement. Make it feel as pleasant as possible, as you remember the delight you had stretching when you were a child.

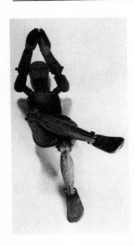

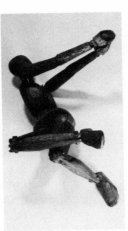

6. POSITION

Leave your right leg crossed over the left as you hold both hands up in the steeple position.

A. MOVEMENT

Exhale, letting your arms and head tilt halfway over to the left, before releasing legs to tilt over to the right. (The arms go first because the upper half of the body is much lighter than the lower half.) Then inhale, bringing both arms and legs slowly back to vertical. *Repeat 5 times.*

SENSING

Notice the full spiral twist of the body—as if two giant hands were gently twisting the lower part of the body one way and the upper part the other, like squeezing the water out of a washrag.

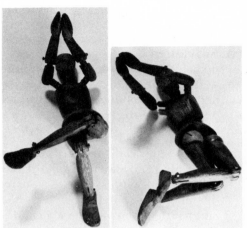

7. POSITION
Cross left leg over the right, while holding the arms in the steeple position.

A. MOVEMENT
Exhale, letting your arms and head tilt halfway to the right, before releasing the legs to tilt over to the left. Then inhale, bringing arms and legs back to vertical *5 times.*

Uncross your legs and relax for a moment.

Now you can put all of this together in a delightful movement pattern:

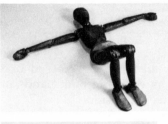

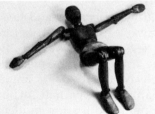

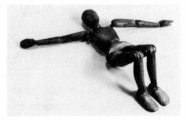

8. POSITION
Leave knees bent, but stretch out both arms to the side.

A. MOVEMENT
Roll the left arm up on the surface of the floor (roll—don't slide—the arm) until the shoulder begins to press down on the floor, while simultaneously rolling the right arm down the surface of the floor (rolling—not sliding) until the shoulder begins to lift up off the floor. . . .

Then, do the reverse, by rolling the left arm down the floor and the right arm up. Do this slowly and gently several times until you get the feel of it.

Now, roll the right arm down and the left arm up as you simultaneously let the two legs drop down to the right. Then do the reverse: As the right arm rolls back up and the

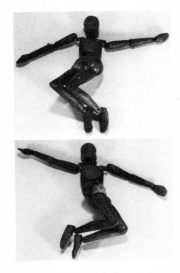

left arm rolls down, drop the legs over to the left.

Continue this movement slowly, back and forth, letting your head join in the movement by rolling left when the knees drop to the right and rolling right when the knees drop to the left. *Repeat 10 to 20 times.*

SENSING
Notice how the entire body twists, stretches, and lengthens. Try to make this movement as pleasurable as possible—like a child, lazily stretching. Or like a cat.

Stop and rest.

Body Image Training
Traumatic injuries cause many individuals to be scoliotic, that is, tilted over to one side, with a spinal curvature. Because this curvature is, in most cases, caused by the spinal and trunk muscles being chronically contracted on that side, regaining control of these muscles makes it possible to correct this curvature.

To test whether you are scoliotic, stand in front of a mirror, close your eyes, and tilt briefly to one side; then return to "what feels like vertical," with the eyes still closed. Then open your eyes and look into the mirror to see if the mirror image matches "what feels like vertical." Is the head vertical? Are the shoulders horizontal? Are your two hands hanging down at the same level?

If you find that you are tilting, then you have clear evidence that your body image ("what feels like vertical") is distorted and your sense of balance has been disturbed.

To correct this distorted body image, do the following procedure: With eyes closed, tilt to the right, then return to "what feels like vertical." If, when you open your eyes, you are off balance, immediately *close the eyes again,* and try to correct the imbalance purely by sensing your balance "in the dark." When you believe you have corrected it, open your eyes again *but do not move.* Did you rebalance this time? If not, close your eyes again, and correct your posture until you think you have it balanced. Then, not moving, open your eyes and check again. If still unbalanced, repeat until you end up balanced.

Important: Under no circumstance should you attempt to correct your balance with the eyes open—otherwise, the sensory-motor system learns nothing and your posture will not change.

After getting the correct balance with the eyes closed, repeat the same procedure, except that this time you close the eyes and tilt to the left. Then, when you get it balanced, do it once more to the right. Then do it once more to the left. That is sufficient for one day's training.

The next day, go through the same procedure again, and you will discover that you are rapidly becoming more consistently accurate. After a week or so, you will find that while "in the dark," you know exactly where your head and body are in space. At that point, the correction of the scoliosis will be complete, assuming that you have also mastered the muscle releases of the first four Somatic Exercises.

At the end, your body image will be adjusted and your muscle control restored. Your internal image and the external mirror image will be the same. This is a classic example of biofeedback self-training—a solidly established scientific method of learning control of bodily functions.

The Daily "Cat Stretch"
In this lesson, the movement pattern of 8.A. is now added to your "Cat Stretch" routine.

LESSON 5
Controlling the Muscles of the Hip Joints and Legs

This lesson allows you to understand why Somatic Exercises must be unrushed and progressive in order to be genuinely successful. You will discover, in your own body, how freeing the muscles first in the center of gravity makes it possible to free the movements of the hips, legs, and feet.

It will also become clear to you how sensory-motor amnesia, by causing constriction of the muscles between the pelvis and trunk, causes general stiffness in locomotion, characteristic of what is mistakenly thought of as an inevitable feature of old age.

You will now begin to free the muscles, not only for walking, but for all leg movements. Many persons who have not hiked or danced for years, discover that the ability and pleasure of performing these activities become, once more, a normal capacity of their bodies.

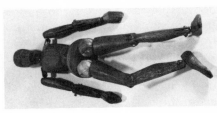

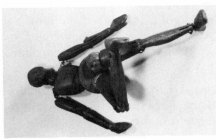

1. POSITION

Lie on your back with the legs stretched out on the floor but with the right knee slightly bent and tilted out to the right side.

A. MOVEMENT

Invert the right foot, turning the sole inward, and keep turning it until it leads the lower leg to lift up slightly off the floor. The right knee will drop down on the right as the foot makes a "scooping" motion upward and a little to the left. Return the foot to the floor and *repeat 10 times.*

SENSING

Notice how the action of inverting and lifting the foot not only causes the knee to drop down, but the left side of the back to lengthen, lifting up the left side of the pelvis. You will discover that the more you lengthen the back and lift the left side of the pelvis, the more you will be able to lift the foot, while dropping the knee.

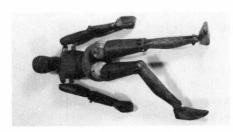

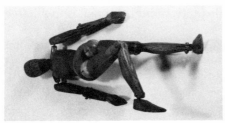

2. POSITION

Now slide the right foot out to the right side, while letting the right knee drop inward to the left.

A. MOVEMENT

Evert the right foot, turning the sole to the outside and lifting the foot upward and a little to the right, while letting the knee drop down more to the inside. Then return the foot to the floor and *repeat 10 times*.

SENSING

Notice what the right hip does and how the right side of the back lengthens to lift up the right side of the pelvis. As you repeat this movement of everting the right foot upward, dropping the knee downward and lifting the right pelvis, notice how your movement extends all the way up into the chest and, even, the neck. Go with this movement by allowing the head to gently roll right as you evert the foot, and see if this makes the movement easier. Indeed, it may now seem almost graceful.

Stop, stretch out your legs and rest, noticing how different your right leg feels from the left.

Now, put these two movements together:

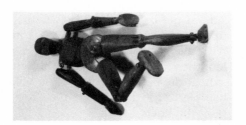

3. POSITION

Have both legs straight at this starting position.

A. MOVEMENT

First, invert the right foot, lifting it upward and inward, as the right knee drops outward and the left

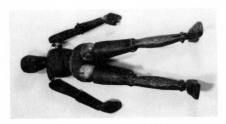

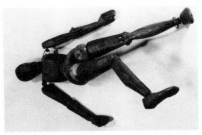

back lifts. Secondly, straighten the leg, and then evert the right foot, lifting it upward and outward as the right knee drops inward and the right back lifts. Then straighten the leg and invert the foot again. *Repeat 10 times, very slowly.*

SENSING
Notice how the whole of the body up to the neck will follow this movement of the ankle. Your body is becoming supple and beginning to move more supplely as a single unit. This is the feeling of synergy.

Stop, stretch out your legs, and rest.

SENSING
Notice how much "more" of a leg you have on the right in comparison with how the left feels.

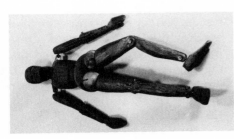

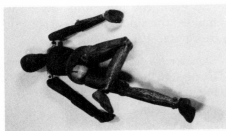

4. POSITION
Lie on your back with the legs stretched out on the floor, but this time with the left knee slightly bent and tilted out to the left side.

A. MOVEMENT
Invert the left foot, turning the sole inward, and keep turning it until it leads the lower leg to lift up slightly off the floor. The left knee will drop down on the left, as the foot makes a "scooping" motion upward and a little to the right. Return the foot to the floor. *Repeat 10 times.*

SENSING
Notice how the action of inverting and lifting the foot not only causes the knee to drop down, but the

right side of the back to lengthen, lifting up the right side of the pelvis. You will discover that the more you lengthen the back and lift the right side of the pelvis, the more you will be able to lift the foot while dropping the knee.

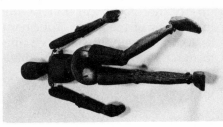

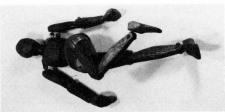

5. POSITION

Now slide the left foot out to the left side, while letting the left knee drop inward to the right.

A. MOVEMENT

Evert the left foot, turning the sole to the outside and lifting the foot upward and a little to the left, while letting the knee drop down more to the inside. Then return the foot to the floor and *repeat 10 times.*

SENSING

Notice what the left hip does and how the left side of the back lengthens to lift up the left side of the pelvis. As you repeat this movement of everting the left foot upward, dropping the knee downward, and lifting the left pelvis, notice how your movement extends all the way up into the chest, and even the neck. Go with this movement, by allowing the head to gently roll left as you evert the foot, and see if this makes the movement easier and more graceful.

Stop, stretch out your legs and rest, noticing whether the left leg is already feeling changed.

Now put these two movements together:

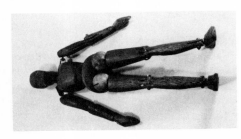

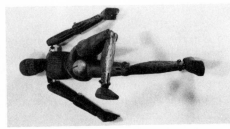

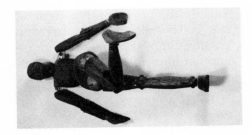

6. POSITION
Have both legs straight at the beginning.

A. MOVEMENT
First invert the left foot, lifting it upward and inward as the left knee drops outward and the left back lifts. Secondly, straighten the leg and then evert the left foot, lifting it upward and outward as the left knee drops inward and the left back lifts. Then, straighten the leg and invert the foot again. *Repeat 10 times,* very slowly.

SENSING
Again, notice how the whole of the body up to the neck will follow this ankle movement. Relax the neck and chest, and your head will automatically rotate right then left as you invert and then evert.

Stop, stretch out your legs, and rest.

SENSING
Notice that the left leg has caught up with the right leg in its feeling of fullness and aliveness.

Now use both legs simultaneously:

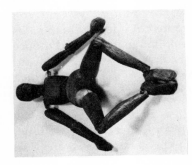

7. POSITION
Continue lying on your back with the legs stretched out on the floor.

A. MOVEMENT
Invert both feet simultaneously, letting the knees fall outward in a "bow-legged" position; then, straighten the legs, and turn both feet into eversion, and the knees will fall inward in a "knock-kneed"

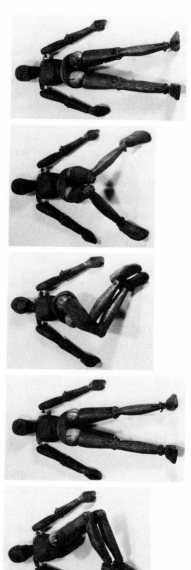

position. Go back and forth *10 times.*

SENSING
Notice that when you are "bow-legged," the lower back tends to arch up into a swayback. When you are "knock-kneed," the lower back tends to flatten downward.

Stop and rest.

B. MOVEMENT
Keep the legs close together, and invert the right foot while everting the left (the knees will drop to the right). Straighten the legs, and then evert the right foot while inverting the left. (Keep the knees together as they drop to the left.) Go back and forth *10 times.*

SENSING
This is the movement pattern of skiing: The soles of the feet remain parallel, while the hips and back rotate left and right. Notice the suppleness of your body as you go back and forth.

Stop, stretch out, and relax.

SENSING
Notice how fully alive your legs now feel. From the point of view of your sensory-motor system, you have "more" of a leg on both sides than you had before. And notice how this aliveness extends upward into the whole of your body, which is now more relaxed than ever.

The Daily "Cat Stretch"
This lesson adds the following movement patterns to your "Cat Stretch" routine: 3.A. and 6.A.; then 7.A. ("bow-legged" and "knock-kneed" positions) and 7.B. ("skiing" movements).

LESSON 6
Controlling the Muscles of the Neck and Shoulders

This fascinating Somatic Exercise, which was invented by my teacher, Dr. Moshe Feldenkrais, lets you discover how the act of paying attention to the movements of different parts of your body frees these parts to move more easily. No better example could be found of how sensory awareness can awaken motor control.

During this lesson, you will also discover that, whereas traditional body exercises make the muscles stronger, Somatic Exercises make the brain more intelligent in sensing and controlling the muscles. It is the inner change in brain function that makes possible outer change in muscle function.

When you have completed learning this left-turning rotational pattern, repeat the pattern on the right side, so that both hemispheres of the brain are completely reprogrammed.

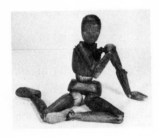

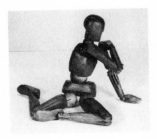

1. POSITION

Sit on the floor with both knees bent and tilted over to the left onto the floor. Place the sole of the left foot against the thigh of the right leg. Extend the left arm downward to the floor at your side, leaning on it only slightly. Keep your torso erect, without leaning your weight back too far. Now, finally, place the palm of your right hand on your left shoulder.

A. MOVEMENT

Very slowly, turn your whole torso to the left, rotating the eyes, head, shoulder, elbow, and torso as far as is comfortable. When you have reached your limit of turning, reverse the movement and come back to the front. *Repeat this 5 times*, then put down your hand to rest a brief moment.

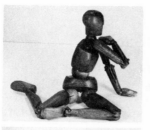

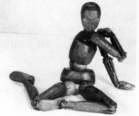

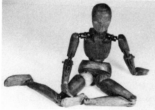

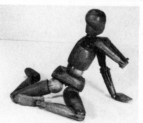

B. MOVEMENT

Once again turn the whole torso to the left, this time stopping when you have reached the limit of your rotation. Stay at this position, and take notice of the exact direction in which your nose is pointing by remembering a particular spot on the wall. (Don't forget this spot, because you will be checking it later on to test your progress.)

Now, holding the torso in this rotated position, *turn the head only back to the right and then, again, to the left, 5 times.*

After 5 repetitions, return to the center and bring the hand down to your lap and rest while sitting. Do not lean too heavily on your left arm.

C. MOVEMENT

Again, place your right hand on your left shoulder and rotate your head and torso all the way around to the left, stopping when you reach your limit. Stay there. This time *move only your eyes back to the right and then return 5 times.*

Return to center, put down your hand, and rest.

SENSING

As you moved the eyes, alone, back to the right, did you notice any trembling of your neck muscles, as if they were trying to move? This comes from the learned habit we have of usually moving the head and eyes together. For some persons, it is difficult, at first, to prevent this slight movement in the neck. Later on, it will disappear with practice.

D. MOVEMENT

Now, do a test, by *closing the eyes*, placing your right hand on your shoulder, and, once more, rotating the eyes, head, shoulder, and torso around to the left *5 times*, each time going to the limit of your turn. At the 5th turn, stop at your limit, *open your eyes*, and check to see if your nose is pointing at a spot on the wall *farther* than the original checkpoint. If you are rotating farther, remember that it is not because of forcing the muscles but of becoming internally more aware of their different functions.

E. MOVEMENT

Again, place the right hand on the left shoulder and slowly rotate around to your new limit *10 times*.

SENSING

While doing this, notice what your *right hip* is doing: It tries to *lift up* each time you turn left, then it drops back down when you return to center. Let your awareness help the right hip to do what it wants to do: let it rise as far as it wants, and you will notice how this improves the movement.

On your last turn, stop and check your point on the wall to see if you have now turned even farther to the left.

Stop, stretch out on your back, and rest for a full minute. While resting, you might gently roll your head

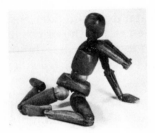

back and forth a few times to see if it rolls more easily to the left than the right.

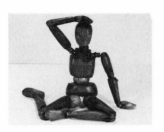

2. POSITION
Resume same position, sitting on the floor with bent knees dropped down to the left, the sole of the left foot against the right thigh, while gently leaning on the extended left arm.

Now place your right hand on top of your head, lightly gripping the skull. Completely relax your neck, so that the movement is done purely by the right hand.

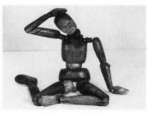

A. MOVEMENT
Slowly and gently pull the head over toward the right shoulder and then push the head in the opposite direction over toward the left shoulder. Continue doing this, *repeating 10 times.*

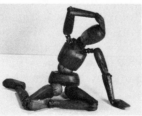

SENSING
When the head tilts to the right, notice how the right ribs compress and the left ribs open up. When the head tilts to the left, the left ribs then compress, while the right ribs open. The rib cage is like an accordion! Allow this alternating rib movement to occur freely, and the head will begin to tilt over farther—not through greater force but through greater awareness.

Also sense that the right waist shortens and the right pelvis takes on more weight when the head goes to the right. The same occurs on the left when you tilt left. Again, allow this movement to occur freely, and the head will tilt down even more toward the shoulder.

Stop and rest for a moment, with your hand on your leg.

B. MOVEMENT

Now do a test again by *closing the eyes* as you place your right hand on your left shoulder and fully rotate around to the left—being aware this time of the movements of the rib cage, the waist, and the right hip.

On the 5th rotation, stop at your full limit and open your eyes, checking your original point on the wall. Have you now turned even farther? You can see how learning new sensory awareness helps us learn new possibilities of movement.

Stop, stretch out on your back, and rest for a full minute.

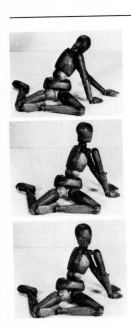

3. POSITION

Sit on floor, resuming the same position as before, except that now you bring the right hand over to the left, to rest on the floor next to the left hand.

A. MOVEMENT

Slowly rotate eyes, head, and torso to the left, feeling how much movement there is in the ribs, waist, and hips. *Repeat 5 times.*

On the 5th rotation, stop at your full left turn, and stay there. Now slowly bring only the head back to the right center, so that the right cheek almost touches the right shoulder, and stay there a brief moment. This is your starting position.

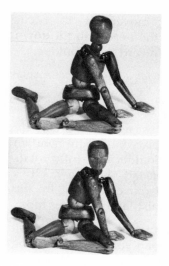

Now, *at the same time*, bring the trunk back to the right center as you rotate the head to the left, your left cheek almost touching your left shoulder and your eyes looking over the left shoulder.

Then, *at the same time*, reverse this movement, bringing the trunk back to the left as you rotate the head back to the right center. Go very slowly at first, until the coordination begins to be smooth. *Repeat 10 times.*

Return to the center after this, and rest for a brief moment.

B. MOVEMENT

Now do a test again by *closing the eyes* and placing the right hand on the left shoulder: Slowly rotate to the left and back *5 times.* On the 5th rotation, stop at your limit, open your eyes to check if your turn is still farther from your original point on the wall.

Rest a brief moment, with your hand on your leg.

C. MOVEMENT

With the right hand next to the left hand, rotate to the left, out to your full limit, and stay there. Now *move only the eyes back to the right* (the head doesn't move). Pause a moment: This is your starting position.

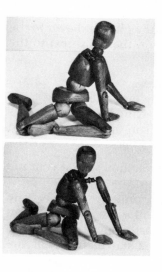

Now, *at the same time*, move the head, shoulders, and torso back to the right center as you move the eyes slowly back to the far left. Go very slowly back and forth, until the original jerkiness of this movement smooths out. *Repeat 10 times.*

SENSING

You will notice at first the difficulty of this coordination—the eyes jerk, and the head wants to follow the eyes. This is due to your habit of always turning the eyes and head together in the same direction. As the movement is smoothed out, your neck muscles will no longer be under the unconscious tyranny of the eyes.

Stop, stretch out on your back, and rest for a full minute.

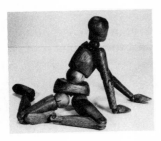

4. POSITION

Resume your position of sitting, with the knees tilted left and your right hand next to the left hand.

A. MOVEMENT

Rotate all the way to the left *5 times* and, on the 5th rotation, stop at your limit . . .

Then, slowly lift the face up toward the ceiling, then bring it down toward the floor *5 times*.

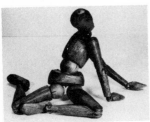

B. MOVEMENT

Stop, with the head down, and then *lift the eyes only* up toward the ceiling. Now, *at the same time*, lift the head as you let the eyes fall downward, then drop the head as the eyes float upward. *Repeat 5 times*.

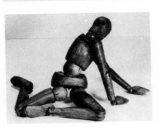

SENSING

You will, again, experience an initial jerkiness of the eyes and a hesitation of the head. You are creating a new program in the sensory-motor section of the brain, so you must go

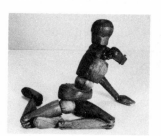

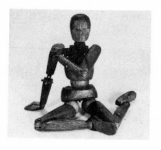

very slowly and pay careful attention. You will, most likely, feel proud of yourself when you have mastered this coordination.

Stop and rest for a brief moment.

C. MOVEMENT

This is the *final test*. Sitting, as at the beginning, with the legs tilted to the left, the left hand on the floor at your side, and the right hand on your shoulder, *close your eyes* and rotate around to the left *5 times*, sensing everything you have learned to sense and using all of your body, so as to achieve a maximal turn.

On the 5th rotation, stop at your limit, *open your eyes,* and check a last time to see if your nose is pointing still farther past the original spot on the wall.

Stop and stretch out on your back and rest.

After you have rested for at least several minutes (or, perhaps, waited until the next day), repeat these very same movements in the reverse position: that is, with the knees bent and dropped over to the right onto the floor, your right hand on the floor by your side, and the left hand on your right shoulder—as illustrated.

The Daily "Cat Stretch"

This lesson contains the final movement patterns of your Daily "Cat Stretch" routine: Do 1.A. and 1.B. to the left, followed by 3.A. (or, better, followed by 3.C. when the reverse eye movements become easier), ending with 4.A. and 4.B. Then take the reverse position, doing the same sequence to the right side.

LESSON 7
Improving Breathing

Once greater awareness and control have been achieved in the muscles at the center of the body and in the upper trunk, it is then possible to learn the art of deeper breathing—namely "diaphragmatic breathing."

This is a Somatic Exercise of major physiological importance. It should be mastered along with a knowledge of the pathological effects of the Red Light reflex on both breathing and heart function, as described in Part 2.

Although this series of movement patterns is too lengthy to become part of your Daily "Cat Stretch" routine, you should repeat them from time to time. This exercise is a lifesaver. Each time you go through it, you will discover an improvement in your breathing; that is, you will be taking in more and more air with less and less effort.

Each position you take during this lesson—on the back, the sides, and the stomach—has its own distinctive sensory feedback and necessitates a slightly different type of motor control each time. This is because each position is in a different relation to gravity.

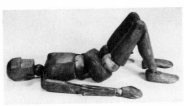

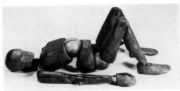

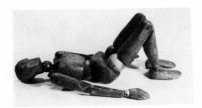

1. **POSITION**
   Lie on your back, with the knees bent, and the feet drawn up near to the buttocks. Keep the feet slightly apart and the arms alongside your body.

A. **MOVEMENT**
   Inhale through the nose and lift the belt line upward as the tailbone tilts slightly downward. (Remember: This is what you did in *Lesson One.*)

   Then, exhale, pressing the belt line downward to touch against the floor. *Repeat this slowly and gently 15 times.*

   SENSING
   Become aware of the upward-downward movement of the diaphragm muscle. It is located at the lower borders of the rib cage from front to back and from side to side.

The diaphragm stretches across this entire area, completely separating the thoracic cavity from the abdominal cavity.

When you exhale, this unusual muscle relaxes upward into the vault of the thoracic cavity, arching like an umbrella, as its elasticity pushes out the used air from the lungs. When you inhale, the diaphragm contracts, making the umbrella shape collapse downward. This pumplike, downward movement creates a partial vacuum, which draws fresh air into the lungs. But be very aware of this: *When the diaphragm contracts downward, inhaling, it must push the viscera of the lower abdomen downward and outward, making the lower belly swell outward slightly like a balloon. Do not resist this natural swelling of the lower belly.* The more you relax the abdominal muscle, allowing the belly to swell, the greater will be the quantity of air drawn into the lungs. In relaxed, deep breathing, it is not the upper chest that lifts, but only the belly.

If, for whatever reason, you hold the abdominal muscle tight to prevent the belly from swelling outward, you block the pumplike descent of the diaphragm, causing shallow breathing.

So, relax your belly as you inhale and let it swell out. It will come back by its own elasticity, and you will not be creating a large belly. "Tight guts" are deadly: They cause shallow breathing and increase the heartbeat and blood pressure. As you take these 15 breaths, let the balloon of the abdomen swell higher and higher with each inhalation, and let it be flatter and hollower with each exhalation.

THE PUMP

B. MOVEMENT

Now inhale and, with the belly round and full like a balloon, *stop*, holding your breath and locking it in. Then, abruptly, flatten your back and belly, forcing this balloon of air upward into your chest, so that the chest swells up. (Be careful: Don't let the air come out your nose or mouth!) Then flatten your chest, pushing the ball of air back down into the belly, while arching the back again.

Continue this pumplike up-down movement until you need to take a breath. Do the movement vigorously and decisively like a piston stroking upward and downward.

Stop and rest a moment.

SENSING

As you rest, breathing normally, can you feel more space for breathing in the abdomen and rib cage? Does the trunk seem less tight? Does everything in the trunk move more easily and softly as you breathe?

C. MOVEMENT

Repeat this pumplike breathing pattern 2 *more times*, being sure you do not let the air out as you flatten the back, forcing the air up into the chest, or as you flatten the chest, forcing the air back down into the rounded, arched belly.

D. MOVEMENT

Now reverse the pattern, by inhaling first *into the chest* (the back remains flat); then shoot the air balloon from the chest down into the belly and arched back; then shoot it back up, then down, and so on, until you must take a new breath. *Do this 2 times.*

Stop and rest.

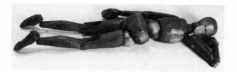

2. POSITION

Turn over and lie on your stomach, with your head turned to the right, and the left cheek lying on the back of the right hand. Let your left arm lie stretched downward alongside your body.

A. MOVEMENT

Keeping your torso loose and relaxed, inhale deeply into the belly, letting it swell out downward against the floor; hold your breath, locking in the air, and then shoot the balloon of air up into the chest, then back down into the belly, and so on, until you need to take a new breath. *Repeat once more,* this time inhaling first into the chest.

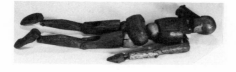

3. POSITION

Change over with the head turned to the left, the right cheek resting on the back of your left hand. Let the right arm lie stretched downward alongside your body.

A. MOVEMENT

Repeat the same pattern, once beginning with the belly inhalation and once with the chest.

SENSING

Can you sense a stretching and opening in the back of the ribs and in the lower back?

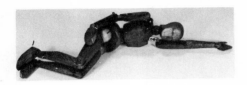

4. POSITION

Roll over onto your left side, with your right arm lying across the right hip and the left arm stretched upward on the floor, to serve as a cushion for your left ear. Keep your knees bent and on top of one another.

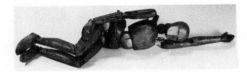

A. MOVEMENT

Inhale into the belly, arching the back and swelling the belly; then shoot this balloon of air up into the chest, flattening the back.

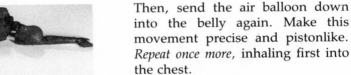

Then, send the air balloon down into the belly again. Make this movement precise and pistonlike. *Repeat once more*, inhaling first into the chest.

SENSING

When you finish the two movements, pause and see if you can sense more breathing space in the right side of the rib cage and waist. Does the right side move more freely? (Remember: Your left ribs are pressed against the floor, so that the pressure of the air is forced up into the right rib cage.)

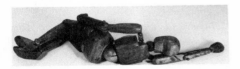

5. POSITION

Roll over onto your right side, arranging your arms and legs as before.

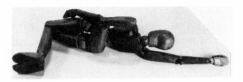

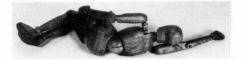

A. MOVEMENT

Repeat the same two pumplike breaths.

SENSING

Do you feel more space in your left side? More ease in movement as you breathe?

Stop, turn over onto your back, and rest.

THE DIAGONAL PUMP

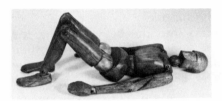

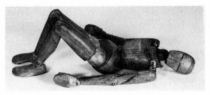

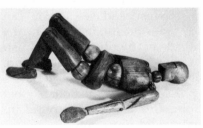

6. POSITION

Lie on your back with the knees bent and raised and with the feet drawn up near the buttocks.

A. MOVEMENT

Tighten your left rib cage, so that the right rib cage opens up broadly. Then, inhale deeply *only into the right chest*, keeping the back flat.

When your right chest is filled up like a balloon, push the balloon of air downward into the left abdomen! You can do it. As you swell out the left abdomen, the back will arch and the left side of the pelvis will tilt down a bit.

Then, shove the balloon of air back up into the right chest, flattening the back and tightening the left rib cage; then, shove it down again. Keep the torso very loose and supple as you perform this unusual movement. It will become easier.

Pause and rest before repeating this movement once more. Try to make it smoother the second time.

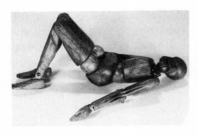

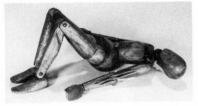

7. POSITION

Still lying on your back, do the opposite diagonal pattern, preparing for it by tightening the right rib cage to open up the left side and by flattening the lower back.

A. MOVEMENT

Inhale deeply up into the left chest, filling up the left lung like a balloon; then, hold in your breath and shoot the balloon of air downward into the right side of the abdomen. The back will arch, and the right side of the pelvis will drop down a bit. Continue this pistonlike movement, until you have to take a fresh breath. Rest a moment before repeating this *one more time.*

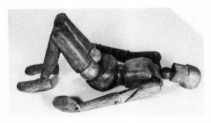

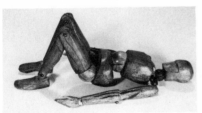

8. POSITION

Remain lying on your back with the chest relaxed on both sides.

A. MOVEMENT

End this lesson by inhaling deeply and slowly into both sides of the chest. Then, hold the breath, as you shoot the balloon of air downward into both sides of the abdomen; then back up again, then back down, and so on, until you have to take a fresh breath.

Stop and rest.

SENSING

As you relax and breathe easily and naturally, notice how much softer and fuller and looser your entire trunk and abdomen feel. Sense the downward movement of the abdominal muscle, as it descends into the lower abdominal area, softly lifting and swelling the belly in full deep breathing. Also notice the quiet feeling of calmness and relaxation that has now come into your body.

LESSON 8
Improving Walking

If the muscles in the center of the body gradually become stiff, the ability to walk is gradually diminished. The pelvis does not rotate horizontally as you step forward; nor does it move upward and downward as the weight comes off and onto the leg; nor does the trunk twist, so that the right arm and shoulder come forward as the left hip and leg come forward (the contralateral walking pattern).

As this stiffness in the center of the body increases, and as a person becomes accustomed to this diminished ability in moving the pelvis and trunk, the art of walking is forgotten. Sensory-motor amnesia occurs, and one cannot help walking like an "old person."

What you will learn in this Somatic Exercise is enormously important for human existence: Humans are the only creatures on earth that walk on two legs with the arms swinging freely in counterbalance. That is why you will find it so deeply satisfying to experience the wonderful circular movement of the hip that occurs in smooth, effortless walking.

In the previous seven lessons, you learned greater awareness and control of the entire bodily musculature, which makes it now possible for you to learn the pattern of "well-oiled," efficient walking. Achieving this efficient pattern will be your graduation present to yourself for completing the Somatic Exercises.

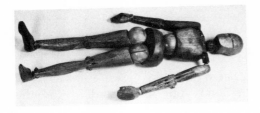

1. POSITION

Lie on your back, with the arms alongside your body, and with the legs stretched out on the floor. Let your feet be slightly separated to about the width of your hip joints.

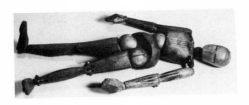

THE VERTICAL DIMENSION OF WALKING

A. MOVEMENT

Slowly lengthen the right leg by sliding the right heel downward on the floor. (Notice that your left hip goes upward as you do this.)

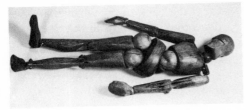

Then, slowly lengthen the left leg by sliding the left heel downward on the floor. (And this time, the right hip goes upward.) Then, again, lengthen the right leg, then the left leg, and so on. *Repeat this 20 times.*

SENSING

As you do this alternating movement, imagine that you are running in slow motion: As one leg lengthens in a new step, the other leg shortens as it touches the ground and receives the weight of the body. Notice how the lower spine curves left and right in response to the foot touching the imaginary ground: The spine hollows inward on the left side as the left hip rises; then, as the right hip goes upward, the spine is concave on the right.

Feel how the large muscles and vertebrae of the lower back adjust to receive the weight of the leg's upward movement, as the foot hits the ground. This up-down movement is the north-south aspect of bipedal locomotion. It is the vertical dimension of walking and running.

Stop and rest for a moment.

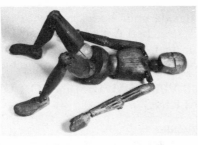

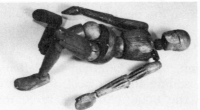

THE HORIZONTAL DIMENSION OF WALKING

2. POSITION
Bend your knees and spread the feet and knees as far apart as is comfortable. Be sure your hips, waist, back, and rib cage are relaxed and supple.

A. MOVEMENT
Let the right knee drop to the left, falling down inside the space left open by the other leg. Then bring the knee back up to vertical and repeat, making sure that the right side of your back rises to allow the right hip to rise. In this way, the knee will go nearer to the floor. *Repeat 5 times.*

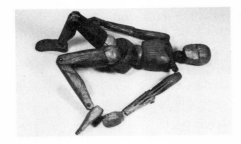

B. MOVEMENT

Now let the left knee drop inward to the right, falling toward the floor. Allow the left side of the back to lengthen, so the left hip will rise. *Repeat 5 times.*

C. MOVEMENT

Now alternate this same movement between the right and left legs. *Repeat 5 times.*

SENSING

As you do this alternating movement, notice how the pelvis rolls left and right on the floor, like a barrel, as the back lengthens and lifts on alternate sides of the pelvis.

Use all of your torso to help in lifting the pelvis as high as possible on each side. Make a large, rolling movement of the pelvis—the torso is rolling but *your shoulders remain flat on the floor.*

Remember this important action of lengthening and lifting the entire side of the torso when you perform the following movement pattern.

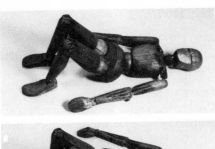

3. POSITION

Remain on your back with the knees still bent, but this time hold them parallel with one another.

A. MOVEMENT

Lift up the right side of the pelvis, by lengthening the right side of the back, waist, and rib cage. *Then, without moving the foot, push the thigh straight forward.* This is a walking movement: The pelvis is rotating forward, as the right leg comes for-

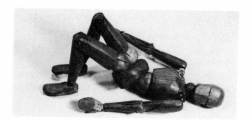

ward to take a step. Push the thigh and knee forward, lifting the right pelvis, *5 times.*

B. MOVEMENT

Then stop, and do the same movement 5 times with the left knee.

C. MOVEMENT

Now alternate the same movement between both legs *10 times.*

SENSING

Notice that this is still the same movement of the pelvis and torso you were doing earlier, except that now the knee is pointing straight forward rather than dropping downward and inward.

You will discover that the more you lengthen and lift the back, the farther the knee moves forward. If you were standing, you would be swinging the hips to take a big step forward. This is the horizontal dimension of walking and running.

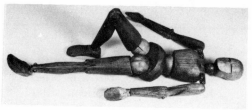

COMBINING THE VERTICAL AND HORIZONTAL MOVEMENTS OF THE HIPS

4. POSITION

Stretch out the left knee on the floor, leaving the right knee bent.

A. MOVEMENT

Push the right thigh straight forward, as you simultaneously pull up the left hip, by contracting the left waist and shortening the left leg. Relax, and then keep repeating this movement, until it becomes easy to do. Then you will be ready for the complete movement:

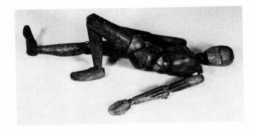

Push the right thigh forward, shortening the left leg. Then slowly *straighten the right leg flat onto the floor, as you now bend the left knee, pushing the left thigh forward. At the same time, shorten the right leg by contracting the right waist and pulling up the right leg.*

SENSING
Stop and clarify what it is you are doing: This is an exaggeration of the movement of walking! Especially notice that the right hip makes a slow circle by rising, going forward, falling, and sliding back. Then the left hip makes the same circle.

B. MOVEMENT
Continue doing this walking pattern of the hips and legs *very slowly 20 times.* One leg bends and pushes forward as the other leg simultaneously straightens and pulls back up. Make the movement smooth and even.

SENSING
Imagine that the straight leg that pulls up is touching the ground, causing the hip to rise from the upward force of the weight; then imagine the same thing as the other leg pulls upward.

Take your time in doing this, pretending that you are a giant, walking in slow motion.

You have now combined the vertical and horizontal movements of the hips, making both of them move in a circular pattern. Remember that the ball of your hip joint is perfectly round. It is designed to go in a perfect circle, once your back and torso become supple enough to allow your hip to do so.

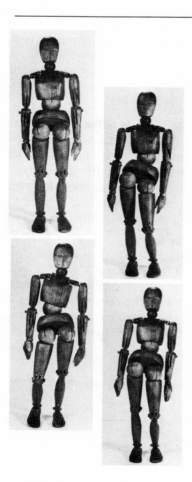

5. POSITION
Now stand up, with your feet directly under your two hip joints.

A. MOVEMENT
Hold the right knee straight, as you allow the left knee to bend, which will cause your left hip to drop down and your right hip to slide partially to the side. All of your weight is resting on your right leg as you do this.

B. MOVEMENT
Now do the reverse: Straighten the left knee, relaxing the right knee so that it bends. This will cause your right hip to drop down and your left hip to slide to the left. All of your weight has now been transferred to the left leg.

C. MOVEMENT
Again, straighten the right knee, allowing the left knee to relax and bend; then straighten the left knee, allowing the right knee to relax and bend. Continue this weight transfer movement smoothly and evenly *20 times.*

SENSING
Notice the circling of the hips in the full movement of efficient walking. The straight leg, by holding your weight, will naturally slide outward and upward, making the lower spine curve in on that side. Keep your spine supple, so that its participation in the movement is easy and smooth.

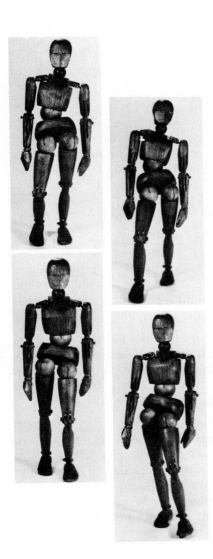

Do not be ashamed of moving your hips freely. At first, the movement feels embarrassingly free, but if you look at yourself in a mirror as you do it, you will see that it is not exaggerated, but is actually graceful. If this free, efficient movement seems, at first, exaggerated, it is because you have *forgotten* what efficient walking feels like. You will soon become used to it, and in your normal walking will have just exactly the amount of natural movement that is proper to your skeletal structure.

D. MOVEMENT

Stop with your weight on the left leg and bring your right knee forward. Then, sliding the right foot forward on the floor, take a small step. As you do so, let your weight transfer over to your straight right knee, allowing the right hip to relax, sliding outward to the side. The left knee now bends. Bring it forward, sliding the left foot forward on the floor, to take a small step. The left knee straightens as it receives the weight, and the left hip will slide a little out to the side.

SENSING

If the knee is straight, you can relax all of your weight on that leg. And, as soon as you do so, the hip responds by sliding out to the side. *Let it slide all the way, until it stops. The ligaments and muscles of the hip will hold all your weight without any effort on your part.* Relax all of your weight on this solid support.

As you begin to make use of this automatic locking of the knee and hip

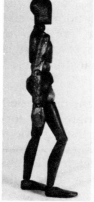

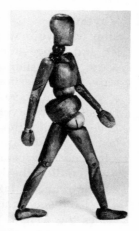

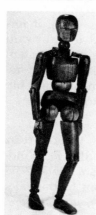

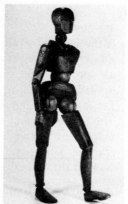

joint, you will notice that the effort of walking is greatly reduced—walking becomes easy, because you are using the bones and ligamental structure to hold your weight, rather than unconsciously contracted muscles.

Practice this movement until it is as smooth as a lion's gait: The pelvis and hips move freely as the weight shifts from one side to the other, but the head and upper trunk remain quietly stable and in balance.

E. MOVEMENT

Now emphasize the horizontal swing of the hips by stopping, with your weight on the straightened left leg, and then bring the right side of the pelvis forward by lengthening and rotating the back—just as you had been doing on the floor, earlier.

Now, with the pelvis brought forward, let the right knee and foot also come straight forward, your weight relaxing down on that straight leg and the right hip moving out to the side.

Next, bring the left pelvis forward, with the left knee and foot coming straight ahead to take a step, and the left knee then straightening to take the weight, and so on.

SENSING

Be sure that, as your right hip and leg go forward, you do not unconsciously bring the right shoulder forward. Instead, pull the right shoulder backward slightly, as the right hip goes forward. When the left hip goes forward, pull back the left shoulder. As you do this, you will feel a supple twist occurring in the middle of your trunk. This is the feeling of the contralateral walking pattern—it is the feeling of free, youthful walking!

You will also notice that this relaxed movement of the hips takes the shock out of the foot's contact with the floor: that is, there is no "fighting against gravity" on the part of the foot, ankle, knee, hip, or pelvis—they can accept the weight, because it is absorbed and cushioned by the springlike movements of the large vertebrae and muscles of the lower back, as they rotate left and right.

References

Introduction
1. Lake, Bernard. "Functional Integration: A Literal Position Statement." *Somatics* 4 (2), Spring-Summer 1983, p. 13.
2. Researchers in gerontology have finally begun to recognize that humans age in very different ways: "Usual" aging moves toward decrepitude, but some people "successfully" age and maintain their functions undiminished. See John W. Rowe and Robert L. Kahn. "Human Aging: Usual and successful." *Science* 237 (July 10, 1987), pp. 143–149.

Chapter 2
1. Barlow, Wilfred. *The Alexander Technique.* New York: Knopf, 1973, p. 110.
2. Basmajian, J. V. *Muscles Alive: Their Functions Revealed by Electromyography.* Baltimore: Williams & Wilkins, 1979, p. 81.
3. Budzynski, Thomas H. "Brain lateralization and rescripting." *Somatics* 3(2) (Spring, 1981) pp. 4 ff.

Chapter 4
1. Kapandji, I. A. *The Physiology of the Joints,* Vol. III, *The Trunk and Vertebral Column.* New York: Churchill Livingstone, 1974, pp. 118–119.
2. MacLean, Paul. "Studies in the limbic system (visceral brain) and their bearing on psychological problems." In Wittkower and Cleghorn (Eds.), *Research Developments in Psychosomatic Medicine.* Philadelphia: Lippincott, 1954, pp. 101–125.

Chapter 6
1. Palmore, E. (Ed.). *Normal Aging, Vol. II, Reports from the Duke Longitudinal Studies.* Durham, N. C.: Duke University Press, 1974.
2. DeVries, H. A. "Physiological effects of an exercise training regimen upon men aged 52–88." *Journal of Gerontology* 24(1970), pp. 325–336; and DeVries, H. A., and Adams, G. N. "Effect of the type of exercise upon the work of the heart in older men." *Journal of Sports Medicine* 17(1977), pp. 41–46.
3. Barry, A. J., Daly, J. W., Pruett, E. D., Steinmetz, J. R., Page, H. F., Birkhead, N. C., and Rodahl, K. "The effects of physical conditioning on older individuals. I. Work capacity, circulatory-respiratory function, and work electrocardiogram." *Journal of Gerontology* 21(1966), pp. 182–191.
4. Bassey, E. J. "Age, inactivity and some physiological responses to exercises." *Gerontology,* 24(1978), pp. 66–77.
5. Gore, I. Y. "Physical activity and aging—A survey of Soviet literature." *Geronologica Clinica* 14(1972), pp. 65–85.
6. Smith, E. L., and Reddan, W. "Proceedings—Physical activity—A modality for bone accretion in the aged." *American Journal of Roentgenology,* 126(1976), p. 1297.
7. Erickson, D. J. "Exercise for the older adult." *The Physician and Sports Medicine* (October 1978), pp. 99–107.
8. Mortimer, James A., Pirozzolo, Francis J., and Matetta, Gabe J. *The Aging Motor System.* New York: Praeger, 1982, p. 9.
9. Ibid., pp. 8–9.
10. Ibid., p. 84.
11. Ibid., p. 6.

Chapter 7
1. Selye, Hans. *The Stress of Life*. New York: McGraw-Hill, 1978; and *Stress Without Distress*. Philadelphia: Lippincott, 1974.
2. Selye, *The Stress of Life*, pp. XV–XIII.
3. Ibid., p. XVI.
4. Ibid., p. 1.

Chapter 8
1. Eaton, Robert C. (Ed.). *Neural Mechanisms of Startle Behavior*. New York: Plenum, 1984, p. 291.
2. Ibid., pp. 295–296.
3. Selye, *The Stress of Life*, op. cit. p. 83.
4. Malmo, Robert B. *On Emotions, Needs, and Our Archaic Brain*. New York: Holt, Rinehart & Winston, 1975, pp. 22 ff.
5. Ibid., p. 58.
6. Ibid., pp. 10–11.
7. Grossman, P., and Defares, P. B. "Breathing to the heart of the matter: Effects of respiratory influences upon cardiovascular phenomena." In Peter B. Defares (Ed.), *Stress and Anxiety*, Vol. 9. Washington, D. C.: Hemisphere Publishing Corporation, 1985, pp. 150–151.
8. Ibid., pp. 151–152.
9. Hymes, A., and Neurenberger, P. "Breathing patterns found in heart attack patients." *Research Bulletin of the Himalayan International Institute* 2(2) (1980), pp. 10–12.
10. Grossman and Defares, op. cit., p. 159.
11. Ibid., pp. 154–155.
12. Ibid., p. 159.

Chapter 9
1. Caillet, René. *Low Back Pain Syndrome*. Philadelphia: Davis, 1962, p. v.
2. Spano, John. *Mind over Back Pain*. New York: Morrow, 1984, p. 9.
3. Caillet, op. cit., pp. v–vi.
4. Root, Leon. *Oh, My Aching Back*. New York: New American Library, 1975, p. 5.

Chapter 10
1. Blumenthal, Herman T. (Ed.). *Handbook of Diseases of Aging*. New York: Van Nostrand Reinhold, 1983, pp. xi ff.
2. Petrofsky, Jerrold Scott. *Isometric Exercise and Its Clinical Implications*. Springfield, Ill.: Thomas, 1982, p. 125. (Italics my own.)
3. Ibid., p. 128.
4. Ibid., p. 129.

Chapter 11
1. Beacher, Edward M. (Ed.). *Love, Sex, and Aging: A Consumers Union Report*. Boston: Little, Brown, 1984.
2. Ibid., p. 313.
3. Ibid., p. 346.
4. Schaie, K. Warner (Ed.). *Longitudinal Studies of Adult Psychological Development*. New York: Guilford Press, 1983.
5. Ibid., p. 97.
6. Ibid., p. 127.
7. Ibid., pp. 128–129.

Chapter 12
 1. Evans, F. J. "The power of the sugar pill." *Psychology Today* 7(1947), pp. 55–59.
 2. Evans, F. J. "Unravelling placebo effects: Expectations and the placebo response." *Advances* 1(3) (Summer 1984), p. 16.
 3. Ibid., p. 11.
 4. Beecher, H. "Surgery as a placebo." *Journal of the American Medical Association* 176(1961), pp. 1102–1107.
 5. Wickramasekera, Ian. "The placebo as a conditioned response." *Advances* 1(3) (Summer 1984), p. 25. (Italics my own).

Chapter 14
 1. An audio cassette version of these same eight somatic exercises, *The Myth of Aging*, narrated by Thomas Hanna, is available through Somatic Educational Resources, 1516 Grant Avenue, Suite 220, Novato, California 94945. *Somatics: Magazine-Journal of the Bodily Arts and Sciences* can also be ordered from this address.

Index

Abdominal muscles, 52, 53, 57, 58, 77
  and withdrawal response, 49–51
Action response (Green Light reflex), 47, 67, 72
  back muscles and, 61–63
  Landau reaction and, 63–66
  See also Green Light reflex
Activity, physiological and anatomical research on aging and physical, 40–41
Acupuncturist, 3
Adrenal gland secretion, 86
Age
  defined, 88, 89
  pride in, 92–94
  viewed as neutral term, 35
Aging
  ambiguity of, 88–89
  and brain, neurological research on, 41–43
  fear of, 91
  and mental competence, 82, 83–84
  myth of, 3, 21, 39, 41, 49, 83, 87, 91, 92
  and physical activity, physiological and anatomical research on, 40–41
  as process of growth, 90
  and sexuality, 82–83

syndrome, 74
Aging Motor System, The (Mortimer, Pirozzolo, and Matetta), 42–43
Agonists, 68–69, 106
Alarm reaction, 46
Allergic reactions, 36
Alzheimer's disease, 84
Andrus Gerontology Center (Los Angeles), 40
Aneurysms, ruptured, 73
Angina, 86
Ankles
  sprained, 81
  stiff, 36
  weak, 36
Antagonists, 68–69, 106
Anus, 56
Anxiety, 55, 86
Archer's bow posture, 75–78, 79
Arrhythmia, respiratory sinus, 57–58, 73
Arteriosclerosis, 73, 74
Arthritis, 3, 26, 36, 72
  rheumatoid, 86
Aspirin, 86
Asthma, 86
Atlas, Charles, 73
Atrophy, 39–43

Back
  muscles, 64, 97
    and action response, 61–63
  pain, 61–63, 75–78, 104

lower, 9–12, 62, 63, 75, 97, 101, 110
  Somatic Exercises for, 101–105
Barlow, Wilfred, 9
Barry, A. J., 41
Bassey, E. J., 41
Beecher, H., 86
Binet intelligence tests, 83
Biofeedback, 86, 111
Bipedalism, 23–24
Blood cell counts, 86
Blood pressure, 40, 41, 57, 86, 106
  chronic high, 73–74
Body Image Training, 106, 110–111, 121–122
Bone spur, 26, 36
Brain, 5, 6, 25
  adaptation of, 33
  neurological research on aging and, 41–43
  triune, 27
  unconscious levels of, 26–28
Breathing
  diaphragmatic, 57, 137
  and heart functions, effects of withdrawal response on, 56–59
  shallow, 36, 52, 56, 58, 72, 106, 138
  Somatic Exercise for improving, 137–144
  thoracic, 58
Buell, Stephen J., 42